CHLORELLA,
JEWEL OF THE FAR EAST

"A Food Algae for a Nutritionally-Hungry World"

by
Bernard Jensen, Ph.D.

PUBLISHED BY:

Bernard Jensen, Ph.D.
24360 Old Wagon Road
Escondido, CA 92027 USA

The medical and health procedures in this book are based on the training, personal experiences and research of the author. Because each person and situation is unique, the publisher urges the reader to check with a qualified health professional before using any procedure where there is any question as to its appropriateness.

Because there is always some risk involved, the author/publisher are not responsible for any adverse effects or consequences resulting from the use of any of the suggestions, preparations or procedures in this book. Please do not use the book if you are unwilling to assume the risk. Feel free to consult a physician or other qualified health professional. It is a sign of wisdom, not cowardice, to seek a second or third opinion.

First Edition

BERNARD JENSEN, Publisher
24360 Old Wagon Road
Escondido, CA 92027 USA

ISBN 0-932615-23-6

CONTENTS

I dedicate this self-help book
to
all the people of this world
who hunger for improving their lives. To those who seek personal nutritional excellence and to those who hunger to live at their optimum level of health.

—Dr. Bernard Jensen

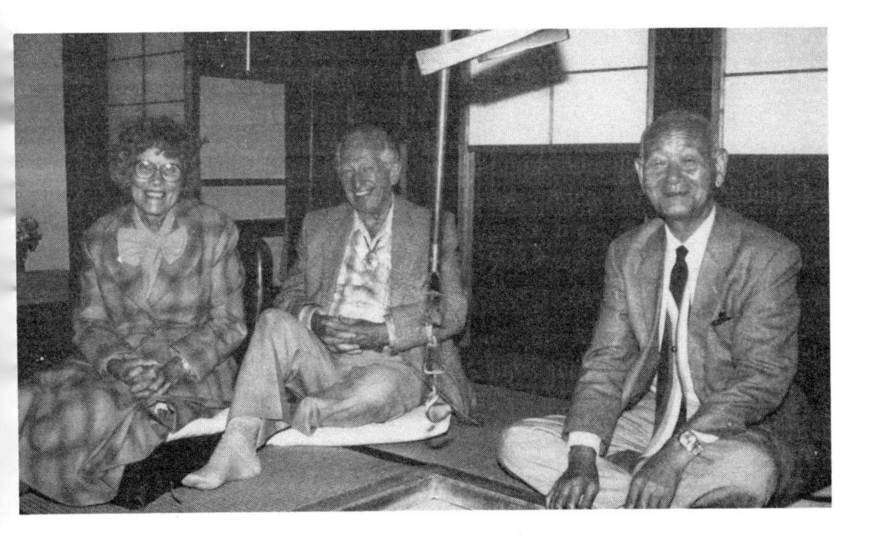

PREFACE

ARE YOU KNOCKING ON THE RIGHT DOOR?

I have never met a person who didn't want good health, but most people are looking in the wrong places. My mother used to say: "If you lose your health you have lost a lot, but if you lose your peace of mind, you have lost everything."

Good health is more than a regular heartbeat and good bowel elimination. Good health requires and includes a positive attitude, hope, creativity, self acceptance, willingness to work and an appreciation of other people. We need all these things and more to be truly healthy. However, without proper nutrition, we can't have any of these.

Without the right foods for the body, the mental life and spiritual life become distorted and out of balance. We need to know this, in order to appreciate the rule of nutrition.

WE REAP WHAT WE SOW

I knew a business executive who overworked himself, ate rich overcooked foods, smoked constantly, abused alcohol and got too little sleep. He had a medicine cabinet full of pills for his ulcers, high blood pressure, headaches, sinus troubles and bowel problems. He didn't realize that his lifestyle was the problem. He didn't realize he had earned each of his health ailments. Pills are not the solution to a disease-producing lifestyle. Some busy executives and public figures add hard workouts at a fitness center to an already overloaded schedule. They consider several hours of intense exercise a week, along with an occasional salad for lunch, to be what they need to stay healthy. It isn't that simple. Health is built up or torn down by what we do *all the time*, not by what we do once in a while.

THE BODY IS THE MIND'S SHADOW

The body follows the mind like a shadow, always coming along, always turning where we turn, stopping when we stop. We make all the decisions that either build health or tear it down. That's why I always say good health starts with the mind.

When you choose to eat junk foods, the body has no choice but to make the best tissue it can with them. If your left knee is made of Aunt Gertrude's pancakes and your right shoulder is chocolate cake, you have to realize that your body is not at fault.

If you choose to watch TV instead of taking a walk, the body is affected. If you take a high-pressure job for the high salary offered, your body will suffer from the effects of stress.

We don't *catch* a chronic disease. We eat, drink and think it into existence.

We *earn* our diseases.

THE BACKLASH EFFECT ON THE MIND

Once we have reached the point where our health is going downhill due) bad lifestyle choices, we find that what harms the body also harms the aind. You can't have a healthy mind in a sick body. Nutrition is not the ntire solution, but it must be part of the entire solution.

Studies have shown over and over that inmates of prisons and mental astitutions greatly improve in their attitudes, emotions and behavior when aey are given nutritionally balanced diets. I consider these studies extremely nportant. When we begin to think of all those outside of prison walls who ren't eating right, we can begin to see where many family and social roblems may come from.

To have healthy minds, we must have healthy bodies. To have healthy odies, we must make the right food and lifestyle choices. It's that simple.

LET'S TAKE A HIGHER PATH

If you can see the need for a healthier lifestyle and balanced food egimen in your life, you know the next step. You have to find out what you eed to do.

Wisdom is "putting feet" on knowledge. Knowledge comes from sitting : the feet of wisdom.

Whenever I wanted to know about a particular health art, I would find ut who was the best man in the field, and I would go and work at his side ntil I understood what he was doing.

The purpose of this book is to teach you how to take better care of our health by sharing what I have learned in nearly sixty years of work ith patients.

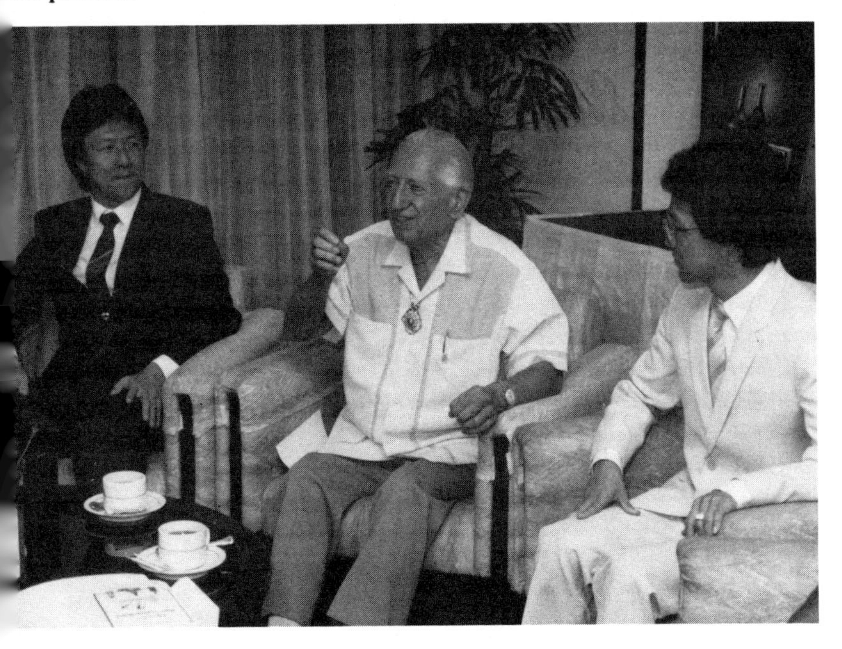

INTRODUCTION

During September 1990, my wife Marie and I traveled to the Orient in response to an invitation to lecture in Malaysia, Indonesia, Thailand, Hong Kong and Singapore, on the subject of Chlorella, the unique health-building alga that I first encountered in the 1950s.

This was not our first trip to the Orient, nor do I expect it to be our last. We have visited Japan and mainland China several times, and I have presented my work to groups of doctors in Taiwan. There is a growing awareness in Asia of the link between foods and health, and a high level of interest in learning about foods that build health—foods like chlorella.

I could hardly believe the warmth, enthusiasm and excitement of the people who attended my lectures. They treated my wife and me like royalty—and they were eager to hear me talk about a food supplement that was of great interest to them.

That supplement is chlorella—a unique, edible, single-celled alga that is rapidly becoming, so it seems, the favorite "space age" health food in Asia.

I'm excited about chlorella myself and I consider it the best food supplement from the Algae Kingdom—possibly the best of the Kingdom of the Sea. So, to introduce you to this remarkable food, I'd like to share with you some of the things I told the audience I addressed in Kuala Lumpur.

There is much to be said about chlorella these days, and I am going to skip over the discovery of how this single-celled food alga was found to have so many health benefits, and just share some of my experiences with it.

When I first visited China nearly eight years ago, I lectured on my work at the University of Canton Medical College. Afterward, I was shown an agricultural commune where 5% chlorella was being added to the hog feed. In raising hogs and other livestock, a small chlorella supplement added to the usual feed brings an amazing increase in weight gain. This helps meet a great need in Asia, where so many people need to be fed. Chickens, rabbits, fish, pigs, ducks, and other livestock raised in China grow to marketable size in much less time. The great thing is, any food that increases the growth rate in young animals will also increase the healing rate in damaged or diseased tissue in animals or people of any age.

Chlorella is a complete food, from 50% to 70% protein, high in chlorophyll, high in the nucleic acids DNA and RNA, vitamins, minerals and other nutrients, and high in the nucleotide-peptide complex that stimulates growth and healing. It comes in tablets, granules and an extract of water-soluble nucleic factors.

This is a food, not a drug, and its many benefits are available to all who are willing to buy it. I am pleased at the many benefits I have seen it provide in my students and patients.

This is the highest chlorophyll food yet discovered, and we find that the "concentrated sunshine" in chlorophyll controls calcium in the body.

Calcium is important in healing. I had a patient once with 13 leg ulcers running green and yellow pus who had been treated at two of the finest medical clinics in the United States without any improvement in her condition. I cut up the tops of nine vegetables very fine and soaked them in water. She drank 10-15 glass of this green liquid every day, and those ulcers were gone in 16 days. This made me a believer in chlorophyll. Using chlorella daily is a wonderful cleansing agent and calcium control to help a person stay healthy.

I should mention that there are other edible algae available in the health food stores, such as spirulina and dunaliella salina. Although there is some good in each of them, they don't hold a candle to chlorella. I call chlorella the the king of the algae. It is the only vegetable food I know of whose activity is similar to that of a broad-spectrum protomorphogen activity.

What I mean is this. Protomorphogens are freeze-dried, powdered animal organs that people use to get the specific nutrients needed to build up and repair corresponding organs in their own bodies. That is, you would take thyroid protomorphogen to provide nutritional support for a weak or damaged thyroid. You would take pancreas protomorphogen to build up a sluggish pancreas. But, chlorella seems to operate on all body systems, cleansing, feeding and repairing any tissue in the body which needs it. Since there are 90 different kinds of tissue in our bodies, counting all organs, glands and tissues, chlorella is like a full-spectrum protomorphogen.

When drinking water wells were found to be contaminated with arsenic in Taiwan, the people who became sick were given chlorella, and they were soon free of all symptoms. Chlorella's ability to remove heavy metals from the body, according to researchers, is due to the adhesion of the cell wall cellulose to the metals, which are then eliminated. This is in the digestive system. In the body, chlorella strengthens the immune system to remove heavy metals by phagocytosis. That is, special, large white blood cells surround the metal completely and carry it out through the lymph system.

Chlorella detoxifies the body and also changes carbon dioxide to oxygen in the process of photosynthesis.

We even find that chlorella has been used to digest raw sewage effluent, producing methane gas, fertilizer, animal and fish feed and industrial raw materials as by-products. There is a limit, however, to the kind and amount of sewage and waste that chlorella can digest. Too much cadmium, nickel, copper, mercury and so forth can destroy the chlorella. We also find that chlorella can be attacked and destroyed by several types of microorganisms, which may have to be destroyed before the chlorella can be used to digest the sewage. It is not a simple process.

I have seen a wonderful master's thesis by Po-Keung Wong from the Chinese University of Hong Kong, titled "Mass Cultivation of Chlorella Species in Sewage Effluent and in Artificial Medium." This is an extension of Dr. W.J. Oswald's pioneering work in the use of algae in waste treatment in the United States.

The chlorella harvested from sewage cannot be used by human beings for food, but fish and livestock can use it, and they can be used for food without any problems.

Possibly the most wonderful thing about chlorella is the growth-stimulating activity of a hormone-like substance called Chlorella Growth Factor. This is the complex chemical substance responsible for the rapid growth rate of chlorella, which quadruples about every 20 hours. Formed in the chlorella nucleus, this growth factor, when taken orally, stimulates tissue repair even in damaged or ulcerated tissue that has resisted healing due to conventional therapy. This growth-stimulating substance will increase the growth rate of poultry, animals and children, but not in adults. It will stimulate and speed up tissue recovery in adults and children. The RNA and DNA (digested or not), together with the available amino acids, vitamins and minerals, supply all the basic materials needed for cell repair.

True healing is not suppression of symptoms or surgical removal of a damaged organ but full restoration of tissue integrity and function. When an organ recovers structural integrity and satisfactory activity, that organ may be said to be healed. Only nature can do that, but sometimes she needs a helping hand. Sometimes we need to supply the foods that nature uses to reverse damage and rebuild tissue.

Of course to remain healthy and to keep the body clean, we have to take care of the lungs and bronchials, the skin, the kidneys and the bowel—the four elimination organs. These organs are able to rid the body of toxic wastes if we take care of them. Chlorella, not surprisingly, is a wonderful aid to keeping the elimination system active and unhindered. Good elimination is one of the great secrets to staying well.

I have to tell you that "feeling well" is not necessarily the same as actually being well. A health survey not long ago showed that 9 out of 10 Americans say they feel well even though 2 out of 10 have a chronic condition. Feeling well doesn't mean that our tissues are not breaking down or beginning to function abnormally.

Most people who use packaged foods or take drugs are exposed to some of the 3,000 additives in foods or the thousands of drugs made from a sulfur or coal tar base. These are not natural to the body, and they all have side effects, long-term effects and time-bomb effects. Some of our chemical additives and drugs have been removed from the market because they are carcinogenic or because they damage the body in some way. We all need protection from chemicals and drug residues that don't belong in our bodies. I feel that chlorella does an outstanding job of keeping our bodies clean and toxin-free. It's like preventive health insurance, taking care of problems before they can start in the body.

Chlorella also has an outstanding record of reversing serious, long-term chronic diseases in thousands of cases. I will include a number of personal testimonies later to show how pleased so many people are at what chlorella has done for them.

I'm sure you will agree with me that it stands to reason that raising the health level and taking care of the body will normally result in a longer life. Put another way, disease and sickness wear the body out and shorten a person's life span. I always found that the longest-lived people I met in my travels to over 55 nations of the world were people who lived a healthy life.

An experiment in the Orient showed that chlorella may contribute to extending the life span of laboratory mice. When two groups of normal laboratory mice were fed the same diet, except for a supplement of chlorella in the diet of one of the two groups, the chlorella-fed mice lived significantly longer than the others.

I have tried to live a healthy lifestyle my whole life. For the last eight years, I've been using chlorella, and I can say, "I feel wonderful." I use chlorella and I believe in chlorella.

I sincerely hope you enjoy my little book. If you decide you want additional details on some aspect of chlorella culturing or its health-building properties, you may want to send for my book ***Chlorella: Gem of the Orient***. It's the most beautiful book I've ever published.

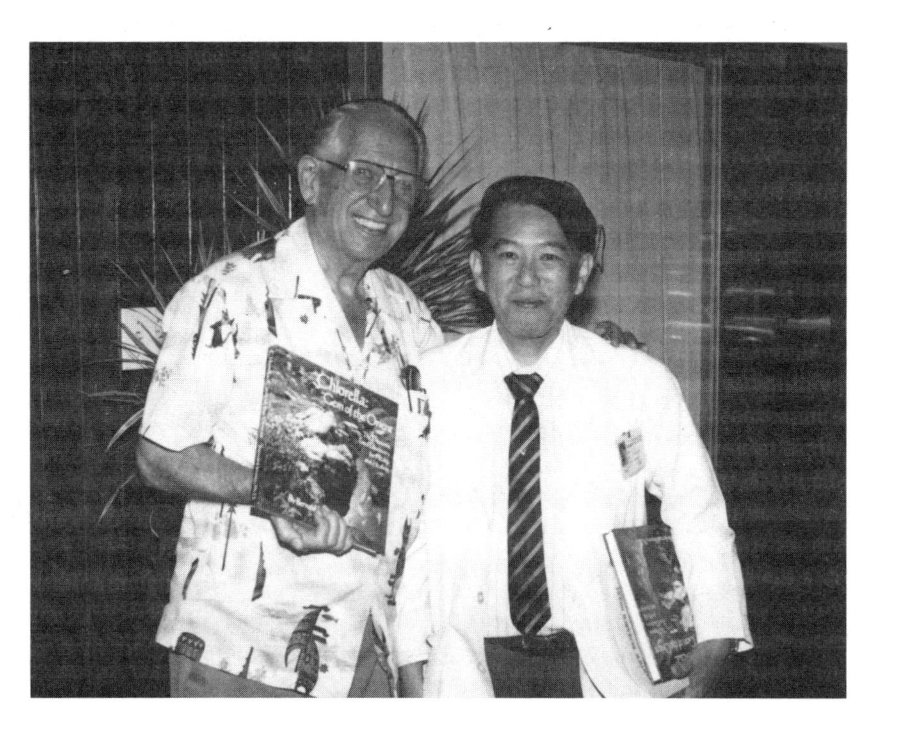

1. WHAT IS CHLORELLA

Chlorella is a two-and-one-half-billion-year-old, single-celled algae that reproduces at one of the fastest rates of any living plant. It is nutritious. It is one of the best health-building foods I have ever encountered.

Discovered by scientists in pre-Cambrian fossils, chlorella has retained the integrity of its original structure through millions of years, which makes it one of the most stable food sources known to man.

I was first introduced to chlorella by a friend in Palm Springs, California. He was growing it in large glass aquariums. It was a novelty item in the health food business at a time when there were many other specialty health foods. I didn't give it much attention until I met Dr. Leon De Seblo, a brilliant doctor and food researcher.

A WONDERFUL DREAM

Dr. De Seblo was concerned about world food shortages and longevity. He was experimenting with several types of food algae when I met him. It was his desire to discover a cheap source of food that could be used to solve the world hunger problem once and for all. He had his own private research laboratory in Beaumont, California.

Not only did he want to feed the hungry masses of the world, but Dr. De Seblo wanted to raise the general health level. He was looking for a cheap food source that would fulfill that goal, and chlorella showed great promise. He was frequently in touch with the Carnegie Institute in Washington, DC, where chlorella research was still in the "cradle" stage of development.

Dr. De Seblo used a considerable amount of chlorella daily and was amazingly strong. When I left his home after a visit, he carried my two heavy suitcases, almost running with them four blocks to the bus station. To me, this showed how chlorella could keep a person young and strong.

Chlorella is high in protein, chlorophyll, pro-vitamin A and nucleic factors that promote healing. It reproduces faster than any other food crop, including rice and soybeans. It is possibly the most widely researched food in the entire world.

Researchers in Japan have found that chlorella specifically helps prevent and reverse a significant number of diseases and health problems. Researchers in Taiwan have shown that chlorella helps clean toxic heavy metals from the body; lead, mercury, cadmium and arsenic among them.

We will be bringing out many of chlorella's benefits in this book.

2. TO THINE OWN SELF BE TRUE —MY PHILOSOPHY

Health has become an expensive commodity in this country because it is so scarce and because it is so hard to get back once you have lost it. The health care system in the United States is a multi-billion-dollar business, and many people are wondering how they can get off the ill-health merry-go-round.

I believe the origin of chronic disease is linked to two basic processes: The lack of needed biochemical elements, and the accumulation of toxic substances in the body. This combination of deficiencies and toxic accumulations leads to a weakening of the natural immune system.

Fatigue, lowered energy and mental depression are signs from the body telling us there is a problem with the way we are living. Our bodies were designed by the Creator to self-correct, to be strong and naturally healthy. Sickness and disease result from improper use of body, mind and spirit.

Proper nutrition, a positive attitude a good relationship with God and man are three of the most important contributing factors to good health.

NUTRITION: WHY WE NEED TO EAT RIGHT

Our bodies are designed to use whole, pure and natural foods. If we stop using refined junk foods, foods that lack nutritional wholeness, and change to whole, pure, natural foods, our health quality will take a giant step forward.

Scientific studies have shown that Americans eat too much fat, and have too little fiber in their diets. Toxic drug residues, environmental pollutants, chemical additives, toxic spray residues and other toxic sources are polluting our inner environment. Many toxins are stored in fatty tissues. Many others build up in the inherently weak tissues of the body.

We need to eat right so we not only get all the nutrients our bodies need, but also quicken the underactive elimination organs to get rid of as much toxic waste as possible.

We can't have pure blood unless we stop introducing toxic pollutants into the body. Without a clean bowel, we can't have a clean bloodstream. My book, ***Tissue Cleansing Through Bowel Management,*** provides valuable instruction concerning proper bowel care and proper cleansing of body tissues. Other elimination channels, such as lungs and bronchials, kidneys and skin, must be kept in good condition as well.

Please understand this important point: ONLY FOODS BUILD TISSUE. We must eat the proper foods in the proper balance and variety to restore or protect our health.

The human body renews itself periodically. The skin on the hands is renewed every few days. Red blood cells are renewed every 120 days. It may take a year to replace and rebuild every cell in the stomach. Because each organ, gland and tissue in the body requires certain nutrients, certain specific chemical elements, we must have the right foods to stay well. We are what we eat.

MY SANITARIUM WORK—AN EYE OPENER

I have maintained several health sanitariums over the years where patients lived on the sanitarium grounds, and I saw them every day. I began to learn that nutrition and living habits were critical contributing elements in health and disease.

When we stop and think about it, we live under constant exposure to germs, viruses and other so-called causes of disease, yet people are not sick all the time and some people seldom come down with anything wrong. I don't believe diseases are caught. I believe that diseases are earned. We eat, drink and work them into our bodies. And if we can work to get them in, we can work to get them out.

My patients often left the sanitarium with a spring in their step, a twinkle in their eyes and knowledge of how to stay well in their minds. I spent a lot of time teaching my patients.

If a wrong way of living can introduce disease into the body, then a right way of living can reverse the process and get rid of it. When there is enough health in a body, disease is crowded out.

How did I help my patients get well? I gave them the right foods to eat, foods that supplied the chemical elements needed to put an end to deficiencies and the fiber needed to improve bowel elimination. I gave them exercises to do, to move the blood, to move the lymph, to quicken the metabolism. I showed them how to do skin brushing and barefoot walks in grass and sand. I taught them about the Kneipp water baths to improve circulation in the legs. I taught them that their attitude was their altitude. I taught them about going to the Great Within.

When my patients went home, they were "independently wealthy." They had their health back and knew how to keep it without depending too much on me.

WATCH OUT FOR INHERENT WEAKNESSES

At birth, every human being is endowed with a mixture of genetically inherited strengths and weaknesses. This heritage is carried throughout life and in great part determines the state of health of each individual. An organ, gland or tissue that is inherently weak may be smaller in size than normal, structurally abnormal, or in some other way changed so that it is less responsive, slower in its functions and activities than normal tissue.

Inherently weaker organs do not assimilate nutrients or hold them as well as normal organs, and they do not expel metabolic wastes as fast as they should. A properly fed and exercised person with many inherent weaknesses can be just as healthy as a person with very few inherent weaknesses. But if a person with many inherent weaknesses is careless with his diet and lifestyle, he can easily break down his body and his health.

The main problem with inherent weaknesses is that they are extremely sensitive to chemical deficiencies. Disease can develop in a body with chemical deficiencies. Once an inherently weak organ or gland becomes deficient in needed chemicals, it can't dispose of toxic wastes as it should.

Toxic settlements and backed-up metabolic wastes create the conditions for a future disease. Inherently weak eliminative organs, especially the bowel, are most vulnerable to breakdown and disease.

HAVE YOU HEARD OF HERING'S LAW?

Constantine Hering was a 19th century European homeopathic doctor who made an important discovery that homeopathists call "Hering's Law." This law states, "All cure comes from the head down, the inside out and the reverse order as symptoms first appeared." This law has been a wonderful inspiration to me as I have tried to understand and apply nature's principles of healing through all my years in the healing arts. Hering's law states in a few words how nature reverses a disease.

3. THE HEALING POWER OF SUNLIGHT

The "sun cure" was made famous by Dr. Rollier at his sanitarium in Leysin, Switzerland, where thousands of people once came each year to sunbathe on outdoor balconies and breathe the pure mountain air. Many cases of tuberculosis were cured that way before the discovery of antibiotics.

There are many ways the sun stimulates healing, both directly by its action on the body and indirectly by stimulating the development of healing nutrients in foods, herbs and plants. The action of sunlight on the skin creates vitamin D, one of the calcium controls in the body. Calcium is required in every healing process.

The sweetness of ripening fruits is developed by sodium, which is why we call the sun a "sodium star." This natural sodium is used to neutralize acids in the body, replace sodium lost by perspiration and to keep calcium in solution in the bloodstream.

CHLOROPHYLL—CONCENTRATED SUNLIGHT HEALING POWER

Photosynthesis is a natural miracle through which sunlight, water and carbon dioxide are used by the chlorophyll granules that make plants green to manufacture sugars and starches. Plants use only the red and blue of the solar spectrum to energize their food production. Red and blue together make violet, long recognized as a healing color.

The structure of the chlorophyll molecule is almost exactly like that of the hemoglobin molecule, except that chlorophyll has a magnesium atom in the center, while hemoglobin has an iron atom. Chlorophyll is said to be the life blood of plants.

From the 1930s to the 1950s, university scientists documented many successful medical applications of chlorophyll extracted from plants. Chlorophyll in sterile water was used to cleanse wounds. Diseases of the mouth, trench mouth and pyorrhea improved after chlorophyll was used. Respiratory infections and sinus inflammations were helped. When rats were fed chlorophyll, their rate of red blood cell formation was increased.

I encountered a woman with thirteen open, infected ulcers on her legs, which had not improved after treatments at two of the best clinics in the United States. I put her on a high chlorophyll intake, using the green tops from nine different vegetables, chopped fine, soaked in water, then strained. She drank three to four quarts of this "liquid sunshine" every day for three weeks and the leg ulcers healed completely.

Chlorophyll treatments quickly faded as the new "miracle drugs" were discovered in the 1940s. But now we find these drugs are not the "magic silver bullet" we once thought they were. Many diseases have developed drug-resistant strains. Some drugs have such powerful side effects that the treatment is as bad as the disease. There are many disadvantages to drugs. In the face of increasing problems with drug treatments, chlorophyll is once again emerging as a cleansing and healing agent *without side effects.*

Chlorophyll is the greatest natural cleansing agent known to man. Chlorophyll not only helps control calcium in the body, but brings down the bile from the liver and gallbladder, assists in the digestion of heavy proteins and fats, increases iron absorption, cleanses and builds the blood.

I have used chlorophyll in lanolin salve for skin conditions. I have used chlorophyll to build up the red blood count in my patients, (increasing the count by as much as 400,000 in three weeks). Chlorophyll enemas have been used to soothe irritated or bleeding colons.

For many years, I have been looking for a chlorophyll-rich food source to improve and stimulate cleansing and healing in all my patients, and I've found that the name of the food is chlorella. This is what I am going to tell you about here.

4. GREEN TREASURE—CHLORELLA

During the early days of television, the "jolly green giant" was a cartoon-like character who encouraged us all to eat a certain brand of vegetables and fruits. In contrast, one of the greatest health discoveries in recent years is so tiny you have to look under the microscope to see it.

Its name is chlorella, and it belongs to one of the largest families on earth. In or near the water that covers four-fifths of the earth's surface are found 25,000 species of algae; tiny, microscopic single-celled plants without roots, stems, branches or leaves. These single-celled plants reproduce by dividing into two or more at a certain point in their lives.

Several kinds of algae are used as food or in food products. One is carrageenin from Irish moss, a sea algae, is used in chocolate milk, sauces, syrups, toothpaste and shampoo. Agar, another type, is added to bakery goods, cheese, candy, sherbet and laxatives.

Far East nations, who depend more on sea-harvested products than we do, have used kelp as a flavoring and food supplement for many hundreds of years. Eastern cultures recognize and appreciate the many healthful benefits of kelp. Their university scientists look to the sea in their research for enhancing the food harvest and health supplements of their countries.

DISCOVERY OF CHLORELLA

The first known laboratory culture of chlorella was developed by M.W. Beijerinck of Holland, a microbiologist, in 1890. Beijerinck verified the algae as edible.

In 1917, a German microbiologist named Lindner, motivated by food shortages in his homeland, came up with the idea of making food from chlorella, which is over 50% protein. His work was discontinued when World War I came to an end and peace was declared. In 1942 another German scientist named Hardner picked up where Lindner had left off, but it took a third scientist, Kuick, in 1948, to complete the basic research.

Because of post-World War II food shortages in many parts of the world, U.S. scientists took over the research done by the Germans. A pilot study at Stanford Research Institute in 1948 showed that chlorella could be grown and harvested continuously in massive amounts, and the Carnegie Institute successfully sponsored the building of a pilot plant by Arthur D. Little, Inc.

The action shifted to Japan as the Kokugawa Biological Institute under Dr. Hiroshi Tamiya, took over chlorella research in 1951. The Japanese pioneered in developing the technology to grow, harvest and process chlorella on a commercially feasible scale. The Japanese call chlorella "concentrated sunlight."

The initial research showed that chlorella had the potential of becoming an unusually valuable food resource. Not only was it loaded with high-quality protein, with all essential amino acids, but it also had an impressive array of vitamins and minerals.

At that point, university and government scientists in Germany, the USSR, Israel, the Peoples Republic of China and England became interested. United States scientists turned back to chlorella, as a potential food and supplement as well as a possible oxygen generator on space missions.

Both the USA and USSR space programs have investigated chlorella's potential as a "space food" and for use in an oxygen-carbon dioxide exchange system.

A GENETIC MARVEL

While the flora and fauna of planet Earth has changed dramatically over the period of its estimated biological history, the two-and-a-half billion-year-old fossils containing chlorella show the same genetic structure as the chlorella of today. This is truly amazing.

In other words, chlorella apparently resists mutation and other evolutionary processes. It reproduces faithfully, retaining its structural and nutrient integrity, and it is genetically coded to reproduce at one of the fastest rates of any food crop known to man.

5. HOW WILL WE FEED FUTURE GENERATIONS

I have visited over 55 countries in search of the secrets of longevity and health, including Russia, China, Peru, India, Pakistan, Thailand, Rumania and Malaysia. I've looked for the best climates, the best foods, herbs, soils, exercises, therapies and lifestyles. But, in many nations today, optimal or balanced nutrition is not the issue.

Survival is the issue, and starvation is the problem. Not starvation in the future, but starvation right now. Most of the countries we call "Third World" nations have large numbers of starving people, people who go to bed hungry every night.

Undernourished people are easy prey for disease in any of the undeveloped nations, just as malnourished people are easy prey for diseases that are prevalent in developed nations.

What can we do? Developed nations need to return to a food regimen consisting of whole, pure and natural foods. Undeveloped nations need a food source that can be cheaply produced in massive amounts, using available resources, energy and manpower.

I am convinced that chlorella can play a vitally important role in the transition from malnutrition to whole, pure and natural foods in developed countries, and the transition from undernourishment to basic nutritional adequacy in underdeveloped Third World nations.

Chlorella is a high-quality nutritional supplement that may be used to increase the nutritional value of such foods as bread, yogurt, whole grains, vegetables and other foods.

Tablets or granules are the main forms we find chlorella in at the health food store. Tablets are fine for the most part—but cooking food and adding the granules to it is becoming increasingly popular. It is all right to take chlorella supplements at the end of a meal, but it would be better to have it mixed in the foods.

Chronic chemical depletion in the body is becoming commonplace in both Western and Third World countries, and the great danger is that people's minds will be affected to the point where they are no longer able to find creative solutions to their problems. The only option we have for "buying time" over the short run is to use a supplement such as chlorella, and I believe that is the best way to go. "Buying time" is necessary until plans can be made to develop long-term solutions.

Long-term solutions would include reforestation to reduce erosion, better methods of rebuilding topsoil, conversion of sea water to fresh water, development of solar power plants, and planning for agricultural self-sufficiency within 20 years.

6. *THE BEST OF ALL*

Of the fifteen known strains of chlorella, the one that scientists and nutritionists are most interested in is chlorella pyrenoidosa. Its nutritional value is high. Its composition can be closely controlled by the chemicals used in the growth medium. Its cell wall is thick enough to protect its nutrients, and its reproduction rate is almost unbelievable.

Under ideal conditions, an estimated 40-50 tons per year can be grown per acre. (With heavy irrigation and fertilization, rice may yield almost two tons per acre per year.)

Chlorella cells are about the same size as human red blood corpuscles, from 0.002-0.008 mm.

COMPOSITION OF THE MAIN INGREDIENTS OF CHLORELLA

Moisture	4.6%
Protein	58.4%
Carbohydrate	23.2%
Lipids	9.3%
Fiber	0.3%
Ash	4.2%
Calories 411 per 100 gram	

There are other edible algae, such as spirulina, scenedesmus, chlorococcum, dunaliella salina and the seaweeds used by the people in the Orient. But none are as nutritionally impressive as chlorella. Chlorella contains vitamins A, B-1, B-2, B-6, C, E, K, niacin, pantothenic acid, folic acid and minerals such as calcium, magnesium, iron, zinc, phosphorus, iodine and the highest percentage of chlorophyll of any known plant source. It also has nucleic factors that stimulate tissue repair and speed up healing.

Scientists say that single-celled algae were among the first forms of life to develop on this planet. They provide the first link in the food chain that makes other life forms possible. This is the ultimate in simplicity.

Chlorella is very high in nucleic acids, the DNA and RNA called by some scientists "the long life factors." Foods rich in nucleic acids provide cell-protective effects, which help to repair broken or damaged nucleic acid chains, thus protecting tissue integrity at the cell level.

The thick cell wall, which so effectively protects the chlorella cells' ingredients, can be broken down either mechanically or chemically to increase digestibility. In fact, the cell wall itself has a beneficial effect. When chlorella is used as a food, fragments of the cell wall adhere to and remove heavy metals like cadmium, lead and mercury from the body.

CHLORELLA—SPACE-AGE ALGAE

At a conference on Bio-Regenerative Systems sponsored by NASA in Washington, DC, Dr. Dale W. Jenkins of the Office of Space Science and Applications had this to say: "It has been amply demonstrated that chlorella can be used in a closed ecological system to maintain animals such as mice or a monkey. The algae gas exchanger has the capability of: a) efficiently supplying all required oxygen; b) rapidly and effectively removing all carbon dioxide; c) removing excess water vapor from the air; d) removing noxious and toxic odors from the air; e) utilizing waste water from washing; f) utilizing urine; g) utilizing feces and other organic and nitrogenous wastes; h) recycling water to provide clean water for drinking and washing; i) supplying food to animals to produce animal fat and protein. The use of algae for supplying oxygen, food and water, and for removing carbon dioxide, water vapor and odors has been considered by many authors for use in spacecraft and space stations, and for establishing bases on the Moon or Mars." As we can see, chlorella may be one of the necessary components for long-term space travel.

OTHER USES FOR CHLORELLA

Food is only one means of transforming matter like chlorella into energy. Because it is so efficient at transforming sunlight into biological energy, chlorella could become a good fuel source in the future. By altering the chemicals used in the medium to produce chlorella, the percentage of protein could be dropped and the amount of oil increased. Research has already been done, showing that chlorella is a good digestant for sewage, producing methane gas and fertilizer as by-products. Research shows that chlorella produced from human sewage should not be used by human beings for food, but it can be used to supplement animal feed in amounts up to five percent. Chlorella from sewage can also be used to make industrial products. It could be used to exchange carbon dioxide for oxygen in many of the industrial process throughout the world.

Research has shown that 5% to 10% chlorella in animal feed enhances the growth of young animals very impressively. Chlorella is obviously one of the most versatile plants on earth, and we can expect to see much of it in the future.

7. SEEING IS BELIEVING

I had become acquainted with chlorella through Dr. Leon De Seblo in California many years before an opportunity came for me to lecture at National Taiwan University in the Republic of China. While I was there, I decided to tour a chlorella production plant.

With a guide from the chlorella plant and an interpreter, my wife Marie and I were given the grand tour of the 16 acres of buildings and ponds where chlorella was grown, harvested and processed in Taiwan.

As we were shown the large, round concrete growing tanks, our guide explained that the company used to water their lawn with the run-off water from the tanks after the chlorella was harvested. But, just the residue of chlorella in the water caused the lawns to grow so rapidly that they made the decision to stop using it.

The Chlorella Company of Taiwan produced two chlorella powders, one for health food stores and one for animal feed. A 10% supplement of chlorella in livestock feed given to young animals, we were told, increased their growth rate dramatically. It had no "growth" effect, however, on mature livestock. The company also made chlorella tablets and manufactured chlorella-enriched noodles. It was interesting to find out that they also made chlorella honey.

Our Chinese guide explained through the interpreter that honey in most parts of the world is now contaminated with pesticide residues picked up by the honeybees from sprayed orchards, sprayed clover and poison spray blown by the wind onto wild flowers. When we eat this contaminated honey, he said, we are exposed to cancer-causing chemicals. So, the Taiwan Chlorella Company kept bees inside a special building and fed them chlorella and fruit sugar, free of any contamination. They are able to market the pure chlorella honey at a very good price.

We were told that the biggest market for chlorella was in the Orient where 3 million people used it regularly as a nutrition supplement. Chlorella is also marketed in the United States, Australia, Italy, Singapore, Korea, Malaysia and Hong Kong.

Most of the research and development of chlorella has been done in the Orient. The high population density of these countries stimulated research into chlorella because of the tremendous pressure to produce enough nutritious food to meet the people's needs.

At National Taiwan University, I met Dr. Liang-Ping Lin, one of the world's top researchers on micro-algae and especially on chlorella. Dr. Lin received his Ph.D. in the United States, and his work on algae was internationally respected. He has published many articles in professional journals.

Dr. Lin's work on the ultrastructure of chlorella pyrenoidosa, using electron microscopes, is considered of special importance to biologists in shedding light on how single-celled algae live, grow and reproduce.

"Why do you consider chlorella so important?" I asked him. "The chlorella growth factor is one of the primary reasons," Dr. Lin told me. "This nucleic extract, when given to people or animals, stimulates the healing, replacement and growth of tissue. This has been proved by laboratory experiments with animals and in hospital studies of human patients."

When a serious problem developed from arsenic contamination of wells supplying drinking water to Taiwan residents, chlorella was given to those who became ill. The chlorella brought relief from symptoms and removed the arsenic from their bodies.

With great courtesy, Dr. Lin gave me a tour of the laboratory where he did his electron microscope work. In his laboratory, I looked at chlorella under a microscope. It was like seeing another world.

In fact, each chlorella cell is its own world, at least until it reproduces by dividing into new cells. Chlorella is a single-celled plant, which means that it grows larger by maturing and developing its own food, but it doesn't increase size by adding new cells as most other plants do.

Dr. Lin explained a little about what he was doing in his work. "With electron microscopes, we are able to magnify up to 20,000 times the size of the object we are studying," he said. "This is very necessary for microscopic algae like chlorella, because the single cells are too small to see with the naked eye, and ordinary microscopes do not give enough magnification to show how the cell is made up."

As we looked at different slides, I began asking questions. "What makes Taiwan such a good place to grow chlorella?"

"The subtropical climate seems to be best," Dr. Lin told me. "In the hotter tropical climates, contamination is a problem. In cooler, more temperate climates, the chlorella does not grow as rapidly."

"Have you compared chlorella with other algae?" I asked. "Oh, yes. Chlorella is superior in several respects. The chloroplasts in chlorella are adapted to rapid photosynthesis, so chlorella grows faster than most other plants. It develops a high percentage of protein and nucleic material. All cell functions are controlled from the nucleus."

"Can chlorella be combined with other foods?" "In the Orient, Chlorella is added to noodles, bread, soups and other food products," Dr. Lin said. "Perhaps the most interesting application is with the lactobacillus acidophilus (the bacteria used to make yogurt). Scientists found out that adding a little chlorella to the growth medium greatly increases the growth rate of the lactobacillus."

"I'm familiar with lactobacillus," I told him. "This bacteria is beneficial for bowel health. Metchnikoff believed that fermented milk products with lactobacillus increased longevity."

"Something in the chlorella caused an increase in the lactobacillus growth rate," he continued. "Oriental researchers found it was a sulfur nucleotide combined with protein and nucleic acid. A very complex compound." "Are we talking about the Chlorella Growth Factor here?" I had heard about this mysterious growth factor briefly during my tour of a chlorella factory. "Yes," Dr. Lin replied. "This same substance has been tested on rats, rabbits, pigs and other animals by adding a small percentage to the food of young animals. The animals' growth rate increases compared to that of animals eating the same food without chlorella. This is due to the Chlorella Growth Factor."

"What about digestibility?" I asked. "Chlorella has a thick wall which has made digestibility a problem in the past. But, we have developed a process that increases digestibility to a very high percentage."

"Have you done any studies on the value of chlorella in removing toxic materials, such as heavy metals, from the body?" Dr. Lin nodded. "We can do laboratory experiments to show that chlorella absorbs heavy metals from water. So, if you use chlorella as a nutritional supplement, it will remove heavy metals, such as lead, mercury and cadmium from the body."

"Pollution is a serious problem," I agreed. "We need something like this to detoxify pollutant chemicals we are exposed to."

"Even honey made by honeybees is contaminated by insecticide residues," Dr. Lin said. "A company in Taiwan is now making pure honey by feeding bees chlorella and fructose. There is no contamination. The bees are completely protected. A large percentage of pollen is protein, and so is chlorella, so it is possible to feed the bees chlorella and sugar in a protected, enclosed environment and get very pure honey."

I was impressed and I told him so. Pure honey is a wonderful thing. In some parts of the United States, the honey-producing industry is having a great deal of trouble because of insecticides. After our conversation, Dr. Lin showed me some of his electron microscope work with chlorella and explained what was on the slides. Some of this work is reproduced on the following page. I am very impressed with the work of Dr. Liang-Ping Lin and feel that the extent of research on chlorella shows that it is both safe and a very high-quality food.

All the following electron microscope pictures are used by courtesy of Dr. Liang-Ping Lin and the National Taiwan University.

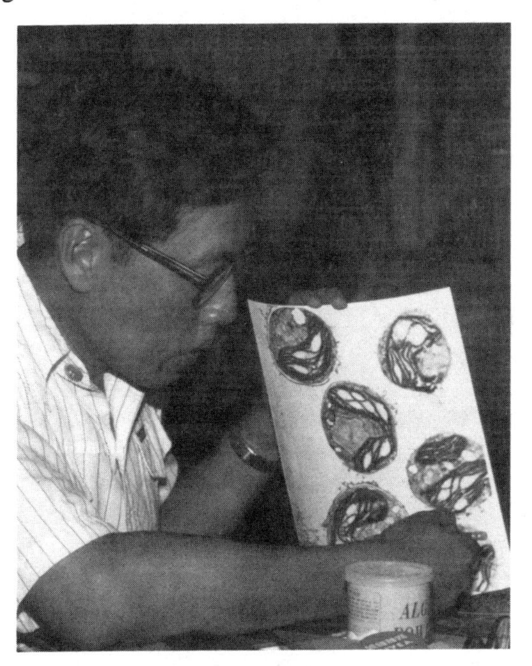

Dr. Liang-Ping Lin of National Taiwan University displays chlorella "daughter cells" which he photographed with the electron microcope at 11,000×.

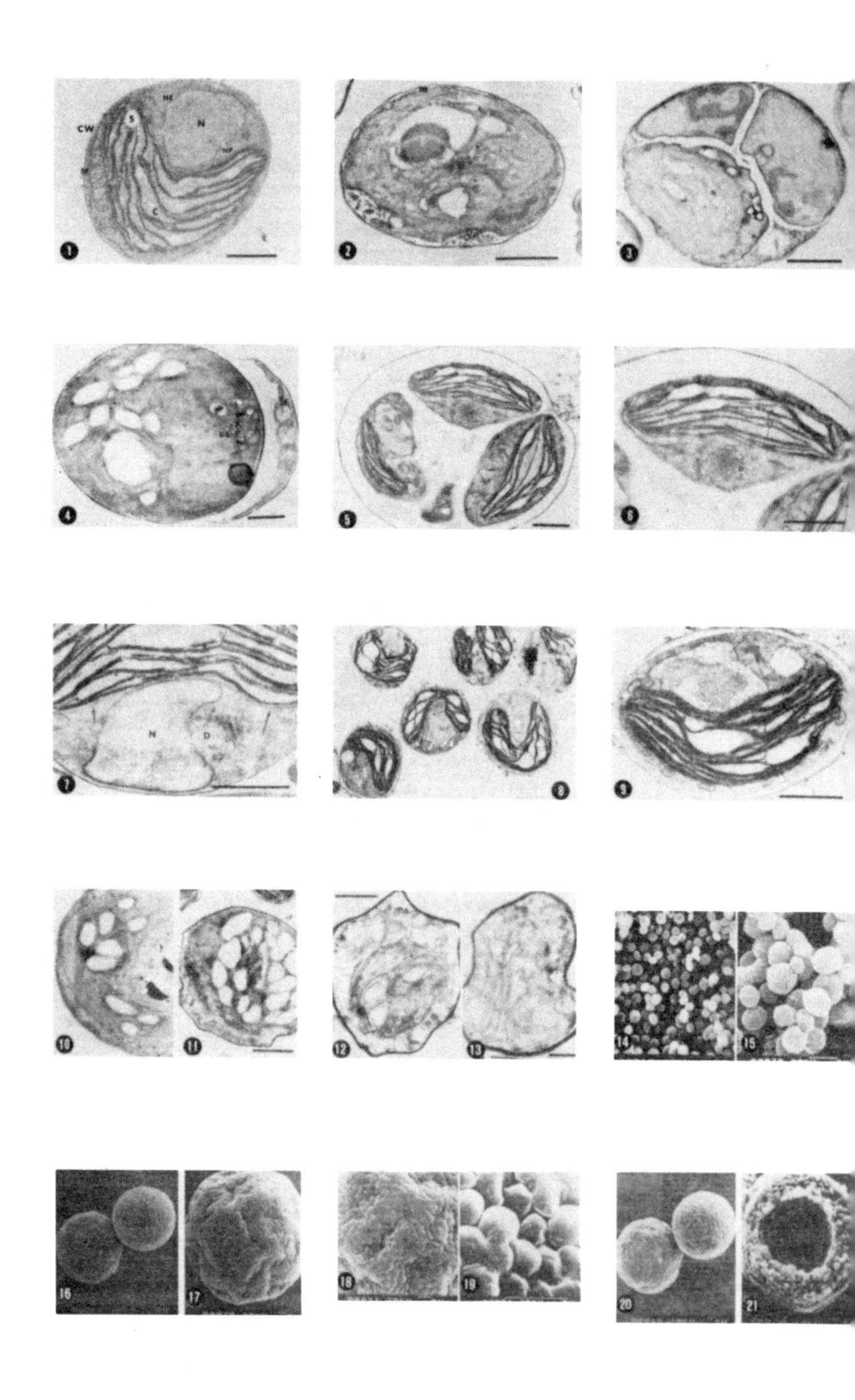
CW
S
NE
N
C
N
D

1. Cross section of a chlorella cell at 31,200× magnification under the electron microscope. The cell wall, which protects the chlorella cell from contamination and deterioration is shown as CW. The cell contains a cuplike chloroplast (C) which holds chlorophyll, a nucleus (N), mitochondria (M) which convert food to energy, and starch grains (S). The nucleus is surrounded by a double envelope (NE) with openings called nuclear pores (NP).

2. Cross section of chlorella cell through the pyrenoid (P), a protein structure that acts as a center for starch deposition. It is crossed by chloroplast lamellae (thin layers) and surrounded by a polysaccharide sheath (starch cup). Vesicular structures (Ve) are shown at the edges of the cell. (39,100×)

3. This is a cross section of a chlorella cell about ready to reproduce itself. Three autospores are shown, each with a newly-developed cell wall. Under ideal conditions, each chlorella cell splits into four daughter cells every 20 to 24 hours. This is taken at 34,500× magnification.

4. A newly-formed daughter cell from an autospore. The chloroplast shows many white starch grains and electron-dense bodies (DB) which are probably made up of polyphosphates. Debris from the mother cell is still stuck to the right side of the daughter cell.

5. Autospores within a mother cell grown in the dark. Each autospore has a large, well-developed chloroplast with many lamellae, starch grains, mitochondria and dictysome. (23,000×)

6. Enlargement of an autospore from Figure 5. Notice the dictysome complex(D) with enlarged vesicles and electron-dense bodies (arrows). (38,000×)

7. Enlarged sections of new cell showing thylakoids (T), nucleus (N) and dictysome (D). Arrows point to double chloroplast membrane. (48,000×)

8. Six new cells showing cup-shaped chloroplasts filled with many white starch grains. Sunlight absorbed by the chlorophyll in chloroplasts provides the energy for photosynthesis, in which starch is manufactured from carbon dioxide and water. Protein formation comes later. The nucleus of each cell can also be seen. (11,000×)

9. Notice how thick the cell wall is on this mature chlorella cell. The first chlorella produced for food was only about 40% digestible due to this tough cell wall. Now, Sun Chlorella company of Japan has developed a mechanical process for breaking down the cell wall and making chlorella 80% digestible.

10. Starch grains in chlorella. (26,000×)

11. More starch grains. (22,000×) Shape of starch grains is much less regular than that of chloroplasts.

12 and 13. Dead chlorella cells reveal collapsed structure and disorganized cytoplasm. The nucleus can no longer be recognized. Plasmolysis—shrinking of cytoplasm away from cell wall due to water loss—is evident, emphasizing the thick cell wall. (12.000×; 13.000×)

14. A scanning electron micrograph showing chlorella cells growing in a pool, magnified 2,000×.

15. An enlarged view of the cells in 14. See how some of the small autospores are still attached to their mother cells. (4,000×)

16. Two particles of spray-dried chlorella powder at 1,000× magnification. Each particle is made up of 4,000 to 5,000 individual chlorella cells.

17. An enlarged particle of spray-dried chlorella powder, 1,400× magnification. These ball-shaped particles are hollow inside, like a tennis ball.

18. and 19. Greater enlargements of a chlorella powder particle show the individual cells in more detail. (Left, 2,400×. Right, 10,000×.)

20. Spray-dried chlorella particles.

21. Spray-dried chlorella particle across section showing hollow space inside. As heat penetrates spray-droplets of chlorella, drying occurs from the outside in, and as the final interior moisture is turned to steam, the hollow space in the center is formed.

8. HOW DO YOU SPELL "HEALTH" IN JAPANESE? C-H-L-O-R-E-L-L-A

After my visit to Taiwan and my conversation with Dr. Liang-Ping Lin, I knew Japan was the place to go to find out what was being done with chlorella.

An island nation dependent upon the sea for much of its food, Japan recognized the potential of chlorella in a way that has anticipated much of the algae's later development.

Chlorella came to Japan at a time when labor-intensive processes were being automated by Japanese designers and engineers, when computers were being installed to control and monitor product processing and quality standards. As a result, chlorella development and technology were worked out in harmony with the latest advances in automation and computerization. Concurrent with this development, chlorella was being intensively tested and researched at Japanese universities, medical schools and hospitals to discover its full potential. The results were gratifying beyond the expectations of even the most optimistic early researchers, and the extensive health benefits discovered gave added incentive for production of the highest-quality product.

The Japanese have developed large-scale chlorella production plants, bringing out a food supplement which has many wonderful health benefits. Just as I have shared all the other health secrets I covered in other countries in my book, ***World Keys to Health and Long Life,*** I want to share the outstanding benefits of chlorella with you.

If we stop and take a brief look at Japan, we find it is one of the most technologically advanced countries of the world. Because of its relatively small land area and large population, the Japanese have had to exercise great wisdom and discretion in using its land and resources for food production. Other countries have known about chlorella—but Japan has made something wonderful out of it. It is not surprising that the Japanese have been the ones to develop such a valuable, highly-concentrated food supplement as chlorella as well as the liquid derivative called *Chlorella Growth Factor (CGF).* Nor is it surprising that the Japanese have had the ingenuity to build more nutritional value into many of their food products by adding chlorella to noodles, breads, soups, pastries, yogurt and other foods.

In the Western industrial nations, pollution, refined and chemical-laden foods, malnutrition, stress and other factors that rob health have contributed to an almost unbelievable rise in chronic disease. Western medicine tries to cope with the diseases that finally result from unhealthy lifestyles and an unhealthy environment, but I feel we should be taking care of the problem at its source. Chlorella is one of the greatest single supplements I know for building a healthy body and preventing disease.

In the Third World countries, disease takes a great toll because of starvation, lack of sanitation and overcrowded conditions. Here we find malnutrition due to lack of food and insufficient variety or balance of nutrients. The industrialized nations suffer malnutrition from eating too much of the wrong foods, while the poorest countries suffer malnutrition from eating too little of the right foods in many cases. Both situations need to be corrected.

Japan picked up the chlorella research in 1951, when a joint grant by the Rockefeller Foundation and the Japanese government was awarded to Dr. Hiroshi Tamiya at the Kokugawa Biological Institute. Japan then continued the research, developing and refining the technology to grow, harvest and process chlorella as a food supplement on a commercially feasible scale.

From a nutritional perspective, chlorella is almost a perfect food. The whole food is eaten because each cell is a complete plant, with all of its life attributes intact. It is pure, uncontaminated by chemical additives or pesticide residues because it is cultured in pure, clean water with nutrients added. It is natural with nothing added and nothing taken away by man, excepting slight nutrient losses in the drying process. In sealed containers, it remains unspoiled for years, and we find that it has only 400-460 calories per 100 grams (3-1/2 oz).

It is interesting to note that fish, poultry and meat range from about 20-30% protein according to Frances Moore Lappe, and while 80% of the fish protein is used by the body, meat and poultry proteins are around 67% utilized. This is something to stop and think about. The protein from chlorella is among the most digestible and assimilable of proteins I know.

In our time, chlorella has appeared as a potential solution not only to imbalanced diets, nutrient deficiencies and polluted bodies, but as a potential solution to the problem of starvation that continues to handicap many of the poor nations of the world.

I don't know of any other food substance that has attracted so much attention from scientists of so many nations in such a short period of time. Chlorella appears at a time when the nutrient reserves in the soils of the world are rapidly eroding year by year, moving toward the danger level. Soils in many countries are already so overworked and depleted that nutritious food crops can no longer be grown on them.

We must realize that mineral salts in the soil must be water soluble to be used by plants, and if they are water soluble, they are also subject to becoming dissolved by rain, washed into streams and rivers, and carried off to the sea. This process has been happening for billions of years, but it is only in this last century that intensive agricultural methods have displaced more natural means of restoring soils. In a few decades, agriculture has stripped the earth of nutrients that may have taken nature thousands or millions of years to put there. Rains leach away more, and we are left with sadly depleted soils. The bottom line, depleted soils build depleted food crops; depleted foods build depleted bodies; depleted bodies build disease.

Because of the world-wide population explosion, we now have over four billion people trying to survive on diminishing arable soils on this planet. Famine may become common on this planet as population growth continues, and we need to look to other means of food production other than current farming methods.

Chlorella, unlike most food crops, is grown in liquid, not in soil. The proper ingredients for its efficient growth can be easily obtained, so it can be grown almost anywhere (climate permitting), and the percentage of its various nutrients can be changed by modifying the growth medium. Chlorella transforms inorganic and organic chemicals into active, living bio-nutrients, sun-energized to provide vital food nutrients.

Possibly one of the greatest benefits of chlorella is its ability to balance the body chemistry. Although nutrition knowledge is much greater world-wide than it was perhaps 20 years ago, food patterns in most countries are imbalanced due to continuing cultural traditions that emphasize certain foods above others. For that reason, I feel everyone should be using chlorella.

Chlorella—High in Anti-Aging Factor

When we evaluate our foods, we use two means of estimating their worth. We analyze the nutrients they supply, and we observe and record their actual effects on the body. In later chapters, we will be presenting a variety of beneficial effects chlorella can have on the body, so here we will look at what ingredients make chlorella the best food supplement of its kind.

It isn't so much the amount of protein in chlorella that makes a difference in our health, but the kind of protein it is. Taking one gram with each meal (5-200-mg tablets) provides only 667 mg of protein, but this includes 29.5 mg of RNA and 2.8 mg of DNA, which help maintain cellular protection and boost energy levels. Dr. Benjamin Frank has referred to RNA as "the anti-aging factor."

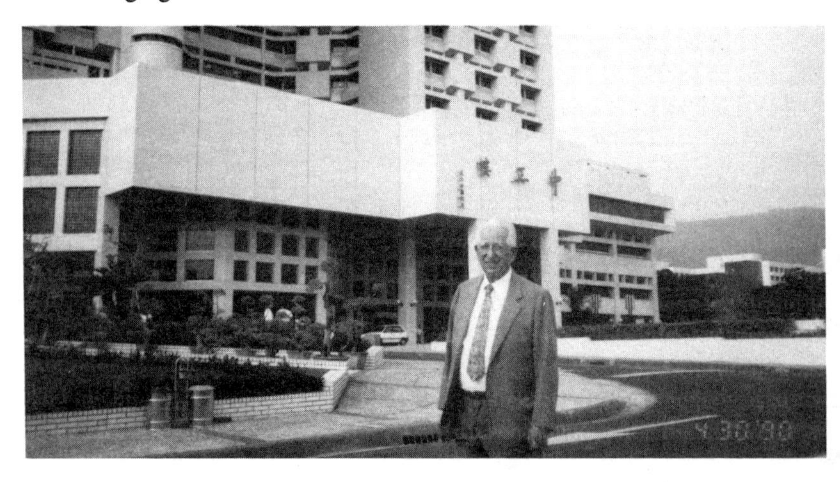

Dr. Jensen standing before the Veterans Hospital in Taipai, Taiwan, where he taught his work to the hospital doctors.

PROTEIN COMPARISON (per 100 gm)*

Chlorella	67
Chicken	24
Beef	24-27
Wheat	13
Eggs	13
Rice	3
Fish	18-29
Potatoes	3

NUTRIENT COMPOSITION OF CHLORELLA (%)

Moisture	4.7
Crude fiber	4.2
Protein	65.9
Ash	7.5
Fat	2.1
Chlorophyl	2.1
Carbohydrate	15.6
Calories 411 cal/100 gm	

Chlorella is, at present, the highest-known source of chlorophyll, with nearly 10 times the amount of chlorophyll found in alfalfa, from which most commercial chlorophyll is extracted.

AMINO ACID CONTENT (%)

Arginine	3.3	Leucine**	4.7
Alanine	4.3	Serine	2.0
Lysine**	3.1	Isoleucine**	2.3
Glycine	3.1	Threonine**	2.4
Histidine	1.1	Methionine**	1.2
Proline	2.5	Aspartic acid	4.7
Phenylalanine**	2.8	Valine**	3.2
Glutamic acid	5.8	Others	11.4
Tryptophan	0.5		

Note: Amino acids are the building blocks for cell repair and maintenance.

---

*Nutrition Almanac, John D. Kirschmann, director, Nutrition, Bismark, ND (1972)

**Essential amino acids.

VITAMINS (mg/100gm)

A (activity)	51,300 IU
E(less than)	1.5
B-1	1.7
Niacin	23.8
B-2	4.3
Pantothenic acid	1.1
B-6	1.4
Biotin	0.2
B-12*	0.13
Inositol	132
C	10.4
Folic acid	0.09

*Daily intake of 3 gm chlorella provides 4 mcg of vitamin B-12, 70% of the U.S. RDA.

MINERALS (mg/100gm)

Calcium	221
Zinc	72
Magnesium	315
Phosphorus	895
Iron	130
Iodine	0.4

Chlorella can be seen to provide a wide array of vitamins, minerals and amino acids, as well as being the highest-known source of chlorophyll. While these are all beneficial, the greatest value of chlorella lies in a fascinating ingredient called *Chlorella Growth Factor (CGF).*

CGF is a nucleotide-peptide complex derived from a hot water extract of chlorella.[1] It is made mostly of nucleic acid derivatives.

Researchers have discovered that CGF is produced during the intense photosynthesis that enables chlorella to grow so fast. Each cell multiplies into four new cells about every 20 hours, and CGF not only promotes this rapid rate of reproduction, but is, itself, rapidly increased in the process.

Experiments with microorganisms, animals and children have shown that CGF promotes faster than normal growth without adverse side effects, and in adults it appears to enhance RNA/DNA functions responsible for production of proteins, enzymes and energy at the cellular level, stimulating tissue repair and protecting cells against some toxic substances.[2]

---

[1]Bunso Rei, ***Health Revolution,*** (Nisshosha Co., Ltd., Kyoto, Japan).

[2]Yoshiro Takechi, ***Chlorella in Figures and Photos,*** (Takechi Chlorella Research Institute, Pub. No. *2*, 1972), pp. 5-6.

Dr. Benjamin Frank, author of ***The No-Aging Diet,*** suggests that human RNA/DNA production slows down progressively as people age, resulting in lower levels of vitality and increased vulnerability to various diseases. Before chlorella was known to be a remarkable source of nucleic acids, Dr. Frank reommended a diet rich in nucleic acids to counter this "aging" process.

Current levels by laboratory analysis shows 3% RNA and 0.3% DNA n chlorella which would make chlorella one of the highest-known food substances in nucleic acids. Used regularly, chlorella would assist in the repair of damaged genetic material in human cells, protecting health and slowing down the aging process.

Nucleic acids in digestion and assimilation are broken down and combined with other nutrients such as vitamin B-12, peptides and polysaccarides. That means that the DNA and RNA we eat do not directly replace human cellular DNA and RNA, but their amino acid combinations after digestion and assimilation immediately provide the "building blocks" for repair of our genetic material. As people age, cell processes slow down. The cell wall, which regulates fluids, intake of nutrients and expulsion of wastes, becomes less functional. Nutrient intake is less efficient and more toxic wastes remain in the cells.

This leads to an increasing acidic condition in the body that favors many kinds of chronic and degenerative diseases. When we have a sufficient intake of foods rich in DNA and RNA to protect our own cellular nucleic cids, the cell wall continues to function efficiently, keeping the cell clean nd well nourished.

When our RNA and DNA are in good repair and able to function most fficiently, our bodies are able to use nutrients more effectively, get rid of oxins and avoid disease.

Cells are able to repair themselves, and the energy level and vitality of he whole body is raised.

It is easy to see the potential benefits from using chlorella regularly. The usual daily intake of chlorella is 5-200-mg tablets with each meal, a otal of 3 grams per day. Of this, 96.9 mg is RNA and DNA, an invaluable aid to cellular repair and restoration. Chlorella protects our health by supporting vital cellular-level functions that keep our bodies fit.

There is evidence that chlorella has prolonged the average life span of mice in an experiment at the Medical College in Kanazawa, Japan. Congenital diabetic mice, fed chlorella as a dietary supplement, lived an average of 2.6 months as compared to an average life span of 15 months among diabetic mice fed a normal diet. Comparison of normal mice who received upplementary chlorella and those who had a normal diet also demonstrated n increase in average life span of the chlorella-fed mice.

9. TUNING UP A RUN-DOWN ELIMINATION SYSTEM

The bowel is the most important elimination organ in the body. It is often affected by dietary deficiencies, lack of fiber, lack of exercise and the stress of modern living. Chlorella has proven itself to be a wonderful cleanser and tonic for the bowel, even restoring the normal function of a flaccid, underactive bowel, in some cases.

While I was at the Battle Creek Sanitarium, I heard the famous Dr. John Harvey Kellogg describe many cases in which surgeries were made unnecessary because of cleansing and revitalizing the bowel. Dr. Kellogg claimed that 90% of the diseases of civilization were due to poor bowel functioning. The relation between bowel underactivity and disease was supported by Sir Arbuthnot Lane, M.D., of London, who said, "The lower end of the intestine is of the size that requires emptying every six hours, but by habit, we retain its contents 24 hours. The result is ulcers and cancer."

More recently, Dr. Denis Burkitt, a British surgeon who did years of research in Africa, found that rural East Africans had no problems with obesity, diabetes, hiatus hernia, appendicitis, diverticulosis, colitis, polyps or cancer of the colon. He attributed much of the credit for this to a diet rich in fiber from fresh fruit, vegetables and whole grain cereals, which keep the bowel clean and make bowel transit time faster.

The average colon contains 400 to 500 species of bacteria, fungi, yeast and virus, which scientists classify as either "friendly" (beneficial to the body) or "unfriendly" flora, such as E. coli, which multiply rapidly until they make up 85% of the bowel flora. These add their own highly poisonous wastes to the colon environment, increasing the toxin level even more. Undigested protein feeds the unfriendly flora. Friendly flora, such as lactobacillus acidophilus, help form the B-vitamins, but they can't compete with E. coli in a toxic, drugged colon.[3]

Some researchers have suggested that septic conditions in the colon, together with various drug residues, form an ideal climate for the production of several types of carcinogens. Other researchers have found that toxins from the colon affect other parts of the body by apparently getting through the bowel wall and into the bloodstream.[4] We have to consider that a toxic, underactive bowel indicates a very dangerous situation.

We can't rebuild a toxic bowel overnight, but we can make a healthy start. There are four components of chlorella that accelerate the process of

---

[3]Bernard J. Jensen, ***Tissue Cleansing Through Bowel Management,*** (Escondido, CA: privately published, 1981).

[4]Clayton L. Thomas, ed., ***Taber's Cyclopedic Medical Dictionary,*** 13th edition, (Phildelphia: Davis Company, 1977), l. 46.

bowel cleansing and detoxification. When used in conjunction with a healthy, natural high-fiber diet, chlorella can do wonders for the bowel. These four ingredients are chlorophyll, Chlorella Growth Factor (CGF), protein and fiber, which work in harmony to clean up the colon.

The chlorophyll in chlorella is the most powerful cleansing agent found in nature. As it begins to detoxify the bowel, it also detoxifies the liver and bloodstream, feeds the friendly bowel flora and soothes irritated tissue along the bowel wall.

CGF speeds up healing in the bowel wall, while the protein in chlorella is immediately available to repair and rebuild damaged tissue, and the RNA so abundant in chlorella also hastens the healing process.

Japanese medical case histories and personal testimonials show that chlorella stimulates peristalsis, activating the bowel to increase the rate of elimination. In Japan, one doctor reported that chlorella has been successfully used to stimulate and regulate bowel activity in patients with injuries to the spine. It works even better, of course, with those who do not have nerve damage.

An experiment by the U.S. Army Medical Research and Nutrition Laboratory at Fitzsimmons General Hospital in Denver, Colorado, showed some interesting effects of a mixture of chlorella and another edible algae on the bowel. The five young men used in the study were started out on 10 grams of the algae mixture per day, which was gradually increased and tolerated well up to 100 grams per day. (They were also consuming about 3200 calories of regular food per day.) At the start, the men experienced considerable gas, caused, I believe, by the cleansing action of chlorella and by the stimulation of the bowel to greater activity. The size of bowel movements in all subjects increased, the dry stool weight in one subject increasing by 400% as the man went from 19 grams of chlorella per day to 500 grams per day. All five men lost from 2 to 4 pounds during the approximately 5-week experiment.[5]

As we look at this experiment, we have to wonder how men having as much as 3200 calories of food per day could lose from 2 to 4 pounds in 5 weeks, unless they were getting rid of fat as well as old toxic wastes. Doctors frequently gave them blood tests, urinalyses and stool analyses, finding no adverse effects from the chlorella. (However, I do not advise anyone to take more than the amount of chlorella recommended on the bottle or package label, unless under the supervision of a doctor.)

In Japan, experience over many years has shown that initial reactions to chlorella may include development of gas as peristaltic action increases. This stops as the bowel becomes cleaner. Bowel irregularity, nausea and fever

---

[5]Richard C. Powell, *et al.*, "Algae Feeding In Humans," ***Journal of Nutrition 75.*** 1961, pp. 7-12.

have shown up in a few cases usually disappearing in 2 or 3 days, once in a while lasting as long as 10 days. Such reactions, occurring in people whose systems are seriously imbalanced, show that chlorella is re-balancing the body. Those who have previously had allergies may develop a sudden rash, pimples, boils or eczema, possibly with itching. This means that toxic materials are being eliminated. We recognize when we start a reversal process that we have to eliminate and take away the toxic settlements in the body that are not favorable for tissue growth, repair and rebuilding. Elimination through the skin and the appearance of rash are generally temporary conditions that seldom last more than 3 to 4 days. The purity of chlorella is assured by testing and approval of Japanese and U.S. government agencies. In all cases, the stool may become green from elimination of some of the chlorophyll.

There are some people, especially those over 40, who have developed a thick mucous lining on the small intestine wall which interferes with digestion, assimilation and peristalsis. For such cases, in addition to taking chlorella, it is often necessary to go through a special bowel cleansing program to get rid of this mucus, as described in my book ***Tissue Cleansing Through Bowel Management.***[6]

Human waste disposal systems utilizing bacteria for the first stage of waste decomposition, and chlorella and other algae for the second stage of digestion and detoxification, have already been designed and tested successfully. I believe that chlorella works with the beneficial bowel bacteria to keep the bowel clean and detoxified, which is one of the greatest needs of our time.[7]

10. VISIT TO AN JAPANESE CHLORELLA PLANT

Finally, a wonderful opportunity came for me to visit Japan, the island nation which had done so much to bring the wonderful benefits of chlorella to the rest of the world.

Japan is made of four main islands and nearly 4,000 smaller islands, with a population of 119 million people. When Westerners think of the Orient, they often picture cherry blossoms, Mt. Fuji and geisha girls, but when they get there, they find "bullet" trains and ultra-modern cities. It is a lovely country.

The first emperor of Japan rose to power in the fifth century A.D., and Buddhism became the court religion in the mid-sixth century, moving in with the native Shinto religion. The Orient has a magnificent heritage in art,

---

[6]Ibid.

[7]W.J. Oswald and C.G. Gouleke, "Algal Production From Waste," ***Preceedings of the 18th Annual California Animal Industrial Conference,*** Fresno, CA 1965.

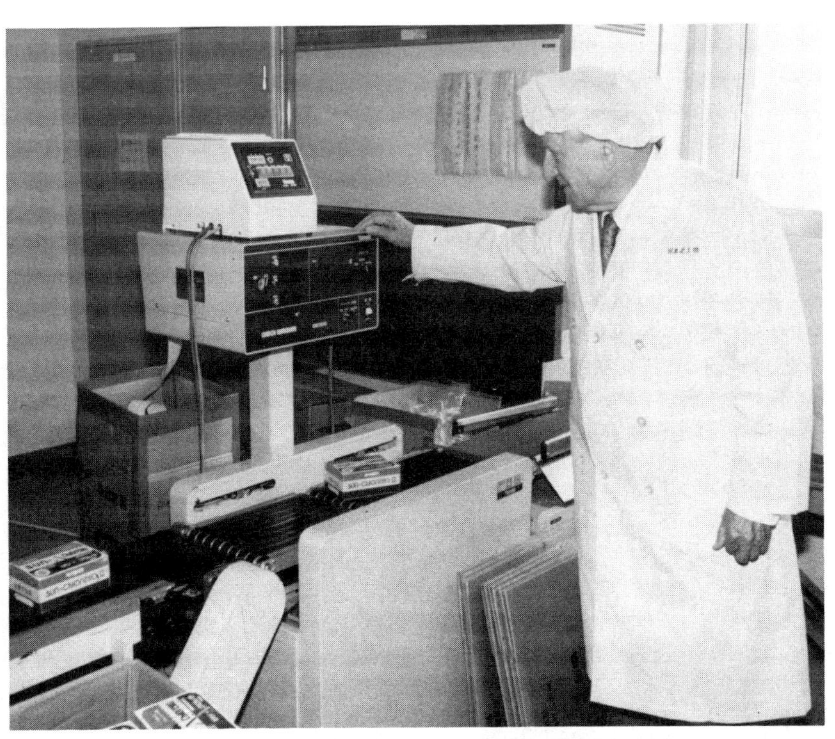

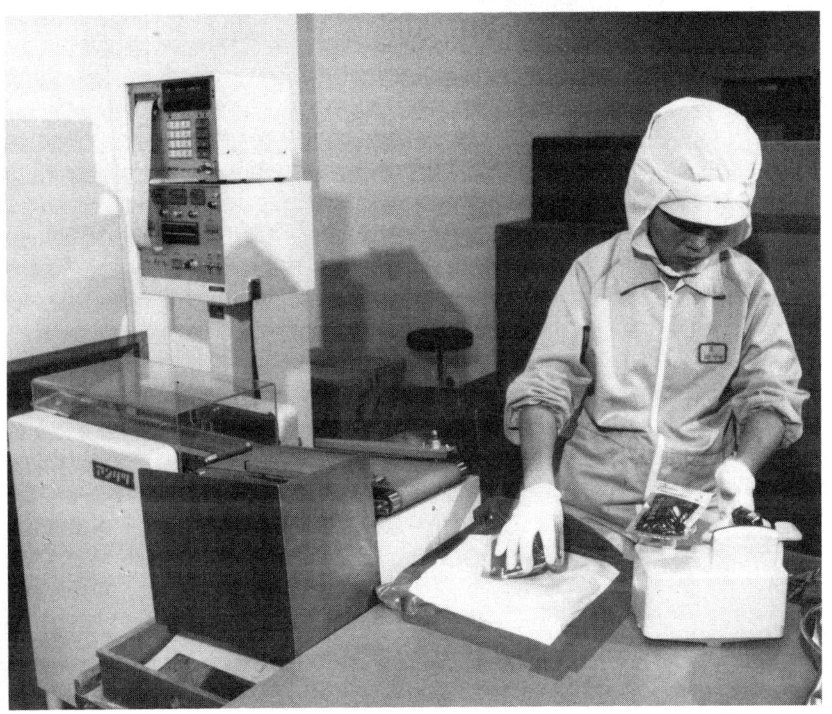

architecture, poetry, literature, religion and many other aspects of culture, yet it is one of the leading nations of the world in high technology and one of the most economically advanced. Pleasantly enough, the Orientals are not only among the most advanced people in the world, but they are also among the politest. Foreign guests are treated with abundant kindness, courtesy and thoughtfulness, as my wife, Marie, and I experienced.

Marie and I first arrived in Okinawa, after making arrangements to see the chlorella cultivation plant there. Okinawa is a small coral island, about 300 miles south of Kyushu, the southernmost of the four main islands that make up the bulk of Japan. Okinawa is part of the Ryukyu Island chain, itself part of Japan. It's hard for many Americans to imagine a country made up of so many small parts. We were taken out past the cultivation ponds to the laboratory facilities, and our guide explained everything very clearly as we went along.

Okinawa was selected as a suitable place for growing chlorella because of its subtropical climate, with an average year-round temperature of 73°F.

We visited the laboratory where the pure cultural strains of chlorella are selected before growing them in larger and larger containers, until they are finally placed in large circular ponds, over 175 feet in diameter.

While we were seeing the plant, I told the guide I was very interested in the ability of chlorella to remove heavy metals and drug residues from the body, and we had a very interesting conversation.

"The problem is, drugs and drug residues need to be taken out of the body, so they don't continue to create undesirable side effects," I told the guide. "I want to know how chlorella does this."

"Chlorella is not like a drug," our guide said. "Chlorella activates the power you already have in your body. The immune system is activated so the different kinds of cells that destroy bacteria and pollutants in the body are able to remove them."

After touring the laboratory, we went outside to the large cultivation ponds. On a pivot at the center of each pond, a large motor-driven steel arm extended out to the rim of the circular pond, moving around the pond.

"What is this?" I asked the guide, pointing to the steel arm.

"The chlorella must be constantly stirred," the guide said, "so all cells are equally exposed to sunlight. They grow faster that way."

We found out that carbon dioxide gas was pumped into the liquid growth medium, to increase the rate of chlorella growth and reproduction. Using the energy of sunlight, chlorella cells were taking in the carbon dioxide and making it into plant food.

Leaving the big ponds with their stirring arms rushing and hissing through the water, we were driven back to the airport. Our next stop would be a factory at Toyama, where we would see the chlorella as it is processed to break down the cell wall.

I had been told that the Toyama plant was where the chlorella was processed through a cell-wall disintegration process that made it almost twice as digestible as normal chlorella. Now it is almost 80% digestible, and we can get more of the good from it. I was looking forward to the trip.

Toyama City is nestled north of Kyoto, at the base of the east side of the Noto Peninsula.

Our guide drove us to the Toyama factory, and we started out in the loading area, where drums of chlorella powder from Taiwan or Okinawa are sent to await processing, the breaking down of the cell wall. From there we went to the mixing or "slurry" tanks.

"This is where chlorella is mixed with water again," the guide told us. "The process is computer monitored. When the mixture of water and chlorella is just right, it is processed by the Dyno-Mill machine."

When the processed disintegrated chlorella was ready, it was sent to the huge spray dryer, fed through a nozzle into a stream of hot air, then dried into fine particles. The dried chlorella flowed through a duct and into large bags for shipping.

Like the other facility we had toured in Okinawa, this one was clean enough to "eat off the floor," so to speak. Immaculate. You couldn't help being impressed by the standards of cleanliness.

Fukuchiyama is not far from Kyoto, the capital of Japan from 794 until 1868, and often called the "cultural heart" of Japan. Kyoto is a city of shrines, temples and gardens—very beautiful.

The Fukuchiyama factory, I was told, was the only plant that extracted Chlorella Growth Factor for use by the Sun Chlorella Company. Of course, CGF is the nucleic material that stimulates growth and repair in disease-damaged tissue, and activates the immune system.

I was shown a large tank where a metric ton of chlorella solution was processed at one time. Clean, fresh water was pumped into the tank and heated to 198°F. Then chlorella was added and stirred, to increase the rate of dissolving the Chlorella Growth Factor out of the chlorella. After that, they centrifuged the mixture to separate the liquid from the solid residue of the cells.

When the liquid is removed, another step in the process causes dissolved protein to coagulate and settle to the bottom. The remaining pure liquid is separated off. Its purity is checked by measuring the optical density with ultra-violet light.

I asked the guide why the CGF had to be dissolved with hot water.

"The heat increases the mobility of the nucleic molecules inside the chlorella cell," the guide told us. "Then they are able to penetrate the cell wall and become dissolved in the water."

"The reason I ask," I said, "is that high heat destroys the enzymes in many foods."

"Enzymes are not the important factor in CGF," the guide explained. "They are important in the green chlorella tablets, but not in the CGF liquid. There is CGF in the chlorella tablets, but here we are discussing the concentrated liquid, where an entirely different principle is at work."

"Then, I would like to know why Chlorella Growth Factor, the liquid, is taken together with chlorella tablets by so many of those who have reported getting rid of serious disease," I said.

The guide considered what I said and replied, "The CGF works together with the chlorella tablet to multiply the beneficial results. The combination of the two is much more effective."

"Can the CGF be used by itself?" I asked.

"Mr. Nakayama, the president of Sun Chlorella, had stomach cancer and part of his stomach was removed," the guide said. "He couldn't digest the chlorella tablets, so he used only CGF. It worked very well for him."

"Yes, I see. Cancer often comes with high acidity in the body," I said. "Evidently the alkalinity of the CGF and chlorella brings down the acidity so the immune system can act against the problem."

"Different people have different degrees of acidity in their bodies," the guide said. "Some need more chlorella, some less."

We finished our tour of the Fukuchiyama plant and went back to our hotel in Kyoto. That evening, Marie and I had an excellent dinner in Kyoto and attended the Kabuki theater. We were very impressed with the elaborate makeup and costumes. I kept thinking about chlorella and CGF—what interesting and useful discoveries they were.

Shiga is located at the western edge of Lake Biwa, northeast of Kyoto. At the Shiga factory, we were told we would see the final preparation process of chlorella tablets, CGF and chlorella granules.

At the other factories, we had seen how the chlorella was grown and harvested, how the Chlorella Growth Factor was extracted from the chlorella powder, and how the powdered chlorella was made more digestible by running it through a machine that broke down the tough outer cell wall. Now, we would be seeing the final steps of preparation of the product for selling in the stores—chlorella tablets, liquid CGF and chlorella granules.

In the Shiga factory, as in the others, many of the production steps were monitored and controlled by computer automation. Technicians and managers stood behind gleaming control panels and computer monitors, checking readouts and adjusting heat controls, density of liquid mixtures, mixing times and other details of production.

The first step in the making of tablets from the chlorella powder was to put the powder in a large mixer and adjust its physical properties.

The mixed powder is blown through a conduit by air pressure into the tablet machine. Tablets are pressed into shape at a pressure of 10 tons per square centimeter. There is no artificial coating put on the outside. Temperature and humidity are completely controlled in the tablet process.

I watched a tablet-counting machine packing 300 tablets of 200 milligrams each into an air-tight, light-tight aluminum foil package with a zip-lock closure and another seal besides that. Inspectors watched gauges as the packets were automatically weighed and checked by computer. Lot numbers were stamped for purposes of inventory and quality control, then the foil packages were put into hard plastic containers which were, in turn, tucked into paper cartons with labels already printed on them.

Each step was checked by computers, technicians and inspectors. The tablets were vacuum packed in hermetically-sealed foil packages. Granules were similarly processed but packed in smaller amounts in tube-like foil containers, which were then put in larger hard plastic boxes the same size as the tablet boxes.

When we came to the part of the factory where the liquid CGF was bottled, the process was explained through our interpreter.

The liquid was measured and poured into the bottles under computer control and the bottles were capped by machine. Caps were washed, dried, then put on the bottles, which are very fancy and eye-pleasing. The filled bottles are then sterilized once again at 248°F. to 266°F., for half an hour. It is difficult to imagine any contamination occurring anywhere in the production process.

Wakasa, Wakasa Gold, and the packaged tablets and granules have been tested and found to keep for five years, so the interpreter told us. Consumers are told to use the product within three years, as an extra added safety feature.

"Dr. Jensen, do you find anything that concerns you in our production?" I was asked.

"Possibly the aluminum foil packaging," I said. "Abnormal concentrations of aluminum have been found in the brains of those who have died from Alzheimer's disease."

"The packaging is in layers," the interpreter responded, "The outside is aluminum, the inside is coated with two layers of polyethylene. The aluminum does not touch the tablets."

I was glad to hear that. Defective product packaging can introduce toxic contamination into food products if proper care is not taken. I appreciated the concern for product integrity.

Now that I had visited a chlorella production plant in Japan, it was time for me to have a closer look at what researchers had found out about chlorella's effect on health.

11. A CLOSER LOOK AT CHLORELLA GROWTH FACTOR

One of the most fascinating facts about chlorella is its ability to quadruple in quantity every 20 to 24 hours, due to its reproduction rate programmed in the DNA of its cell nucleus. Because of this and other factors in the nucleus of this single-celled algae, chlorella stimulates in young animals and plants, and increases the healing rate in damaged tissue.

The almost magical healing and growth-stimulating properties of chlorella encouraged top scientists in several countries to analyze chlorella to find out what biochemical components prompted these wonderful effects.

The story of the search for this mystery factor and the unraveling of its mysterious powers is a fascinating one, but to really appreciate this story, we need to begin by understanding what factors contribute to healing.

In man and other mammals, genetic factors and hormones work together with proteins, vitamins and certain chemicals in the bloodstream to repair and replace damaged tissue. In man, the same pituitary hormone that stimulates growth also stimulates healing. We find that healing is often a form of growth, because new tissue is being made. Other types of healing involve removing toxic substances from the body or remedying nutrient or chemical deficiencies. Tissue repair is usually required in these types of conditions too.

In the 1930s, Browne Landone wrote about what he called "auxins" in young plants that seemed to stimulate renewed hormonal activity in animals and people. Sprouts, tiny seedlings of carrots, beets, radishes and other food plants had an abundant supply of these substances, while mature plants apparently had little or no auxins. At a large urban zoo in the U.S., wild animals which had not reproduced in years were given fresh sprouts to eat. Their sexual vigor and interest returned, and they began to reproduce again. For the average person, we find that appropriate nutritional intake is the single most important element in maintaining health and preventing disease.

12. CHLORELLA IS A WHOLE, PURE AND NATURAL FOOD

Every time I lecture about whole, pure and natural foods, people begin to understand how important foods are in preventing disease and feeling wonderful. They are often surprised to find out how easy it is to understand the basic principles of nutrition.

Most commercially marketed foods today come in a package, can or bottle. The reasons for this can be summed up in two words: profit and convenience. The food industry is not in business to enhance or promote consumer health. We need to understand this.

Health is a *consumer* responsibility, and if you really want to enjoy health, you need to learn some practical things about food.

The greatest thing about whole foods such as eggs, seeds nuts, grains, legumes and chlorella is they contain *all the factors necessary to bring forth new life.* If you plant a seed or a single whole grain, it will grow. If you plant polished rice, it will not grow. Whole foods are the kinds of foods that are best for us because they contain the greatest amount of life factors.

I am not suggesting that pineapple skins and leaves, peach pits or cantaloupe rinds must be eaten. What I am saying is that we should eat as much of each food as possible because the skins and seeds often contain valuable nutrients needed by the body. Whole foods are foods with nothing taken away by man.

Many packaged foods contain chemical preservatives to give them eternal shelf life, chemical colors and flavorings to make them more attractive, chemical texturizers to make them more interesting to the taste, and various other chemical additives. These chemicals are not natural to the body, and even if they were harmless by themselves (which many nutritionists doubt), no one knows what they do when mixed with other chemicals from other foods or whether they will react with drug residues retained by tissues in the body. I am not sure any chemical food additive should be called "safe," and I do not advise eating any food containing chemical additives.

Some fruits and vegetables still have residues of pesticide spray on them and should be carefully washed before use.

Fresh meat, in some places, is sprayed with a chemical solution to prevent "browning" and keep the color more attractive.

Salad ingredients in salad bars are sometimes sprayed with a chemical to keep them looking fresher.

Any foods known to have chemicals on them or in them are at least potentially harmful to the body, because the chemicals may settle in inherently weak tissues or react with other chemicals in the body to cause trouble. *Pure foods are the only safe foods to eat.*

Man was created in a natural environment to eat foods as nature made them, and the human digestive system is best suited for these foods. In our time, there are thousands of hybrid food crops, foods grown from seeds with a genetic structure that has been tampered with by man. I feel nature knows best. The biochemistry of foods is so complex and subtle that man simply doesn't know what he is doing when he breeds new types of food plants.

Seeds are the sex glands of fruit. Seedless grapes and seedless oranges are basically lifeless foods because the sex factors have been removed.

Man has bred many types of fruit and vegetables for larger size, more attractive color and easier picking by machines. This has nothing to do with nutritional quality, in many cases. Again, I feel nature produces the best foods for man, and I believe that the more man tampers with foods, the more food value is lost. Natural foods are the best for our use.

Chlorella is a single-celled algae, a whole food. Throughout its two-billion-year history on this planet, it has survived because its tough outer shell protected its genetic integrity, and it is one of the most efficient foods on earth in using and concentrating sunshine, as shown by its high chlorophyll content and rapid reproduction. *Chlorella is a whole food with all the materials to support life.*

In contrast to soil-grown foods which are treated with pesticides, chlorella is grown in a liquid-nutrient medium made from purified water and toxin-free nutrient chemicals, including trace elements. *Chlorella is free of toxic residues and has no chemical additives.* It is a pure food. Its genetic integrity has remained constant for over two billion years, as fossil remains have demonstrated.

Man has picked out the best strains of chlorella to grow and harvest, but has not tampered with its genetic structure. *Chlorella is a natural food.* Chlorella is not a drug or a medicine, but a food. It is nonstimulating, not a depressant and has no undesirable side effects.

Chlorella is spray-dried at moderately high temperatures during a very brief exposure to ensure its preservation and cleanliness, it is then pulverized to increase its digestiblity. These processes protect and increase its maximum nutrient value.

I have explained why I believe in whole, pure and natural foods, and from this, you can see one of the main reasons why I consider chlorella a "gem" among foods. I recommend it to all of my patients.

13. DO YOU KNOW WHAT YOUR LIVER IS DOING TONIGHT?

When we look at the human body from a wholistic standpoint, we realize that every cell, tissue, gland and organ is designed to support and complement all the others. If an organ is not sufficiently healthy to life and support the others, it drags them down, contributing to the general underactivity that invites disease. Stronger organs, glands and tissues tend to support and compensate for the weaker ones, and this is the basis of many of the natural healing arts. If the whole body is strengthened, the stronger organs may help the weaker ones overcome any abnormal condition.

One of these vital organs is the liver. Not only is it the largest organ in the body, weighing 2½ to 3½ pounds in the average adult, it is also one of the busiest and most important. In fact, the liver does so many things, it is subject to breakdown in more ways than most other organs, and liver breakdown or underactivity affects every single organ and every single tissue in the body.

The liver is a kind of one-man band in the body. It makes a pint of bile a day, some of which is stored. It also purifies the blood by means of white blood cells that line tiny hollow chambers throughout the liver. These protective cells neutralize any toxic material that comes by as the blood flows through. The liver converts extra sugar in the blood into glycogen for storage, prepares nutrients in the blood for assimilation by the cells, and stores iron and vitamins B-12, A, D, E and K. The liver disposes of worn-out blood cells, makes plasma proteins, helps regulate blood volume, takes part in heat production and produces blood anticoagulants. It manufactures some of the lecithin and most of the cholesterol needed by the body each day. (Despite its bad reputation with heart disease, cholesterol is essential to the formation of several hormones, to the nervous system and brain, and to every cell in the body.)

The liver has one of the most dangerous jobs in the body. According to Anthony and Thibodeau in their up-to-date ***Textbook of Anatomy and Physiology,*** "A number of poisonous substances enter the bloodstream from the intestines," and *the liver is the first organ to receive blood returning from the small intestine during and after the digestion and assimilation processes.* Toxins that arrive at the liver may include alcohol, drugs, chemicals from food additives, bacterial wastes, incompletely digested proteins, pesticide residues from foods, and toxins formed in the intestine, some or all of which may accompany food particles into the bloodstream.

Blood enters the liver by the hepatic artery to provide oxygen and nutrients to the liver at the same time venous blood from the portal vein is coming through for "examination," so to speak, loaded with food particles and other substances freshly assimilated through the small intestine. Bacteria, toxins and foreign matter that enter with the food from the small intestine are filtered out by the liver.

Alcohol is one of the most common causes of cirrhosis of the liver, a disease in which tissue is repeatedly destroyed and regenerated until alterations in connective tissue block the liver veins, leading to liver failure and death if alcohol intake is not stopped. Alcohol destroys cells by dehydration, even as the liver breaks the alcohol molecules down into harmless subproducts. Because alcohol can supply energy (70 calories/ounce) and displace foods in the diet, heavy drinkers and alcoholics do not eat much and are commonly malnourished. Resulting nutrient deficiencies in the diet may contribute to underactivity in many organs, anemia, neuritis, destruction of brain cells, pellagra and frequent respiratory infections. During advanced cirrhosis, the liver is so underactive that it is unable to perform any of its functions adequately.[8]

Hepatitis is liver inflammation due to infection or toxins, with fever, weakness, fatigue, discomfort, headaches and possibly jaundice. Jaundice, a condition resulting in a yellow tint of skin, is caused when the bile duct is blocked and bile is forced into the bloodstream.

There are many other liver and gallbladder conditions, but the point is to show that the liver can be overcome by toxins of certain types and quantities. When the detoxification system of the liver is overwhelmed, various toxic materials are carried in the bloodstream to every organ, gland and tissue in the body. Normally, according to ***Taber's Cyclopedic Medical***

---

[8]Gerald J. Tortora and Nicholas P. Anagnostakos, ***Principles of Anatomy and Physiology,*** Harper and Row, Publishers, NY (1981), pp. 616-620, 638, 640.

Dictionary, the liver detoxifies *indole* and skatole, products from incomplete protein digestion that manage to get through the small intestinal wall along with normal nutrients.[9] These and other toxins are deposited in inherently weak tissues of the body as they move along in the bloodstream.

Once toxic materials are able to bypass the liver, the lymphatic system, kidneys, lungs and skin begin experiencing trouble. Excess catarrh may be generated as tissues respond to irritation. In the final stages of cirrhosis, bowel toxins become so extensive that brain function is seriously affected, as shown by hallucinations and severe tremors. Yet, at lower levels of liver dysfunction, organs may still be exposed to toxins without showing symptoms, excepting possibly catarrh and fatigue. We find that many chronic diseases progress slowly and invisibly inside the body for many years before laboratory tests or symptoms reveal something wrong.

Most people are born with a healthy liver, although in a few cases, we find inherent weaknesses or genetic conditions. So, what happens to create underactivity and toxic breakdown in the liver?

The liver not only filters the venous blood, but is fed by the arterial blood. It is the quality and cleanliness of the blood that determines whether the liver functions normally or becomes underactive. The degree of oxygenation of the blood by the lungs affects its activity level. It is the efficiency of the elimination channels, especially the bowel, that determines how clean the blood is that reaches the liver. Nutrient quality of the blood depends on diet, digestion and assimilation. Freedom from toxic matter depends mainly on the bowel.

The health of the liver depends upon what is going on behind the scenes in the lungs, stomach, pancreas and bowel, day by day, year by year. A continuing poor diet and a chronically underactive bowel wear down the liver as the constant dripping of water wears away rock. When the liver finally becomes underactive, the last major barrier to toxic settlements in other organs, glands, tissues and systems is crippled.

With the liver unable to efficiently detoxify the blood, the effects of alcohol, drug residues, chemicals, heavy metals, pesticide residues, indole, skatole and various toxins from the bowel have a magnified effect on the lymphatic system, kidneys, skin, respiratory system, spleen, brain and all other parts of the body. There may be no dramatic symptoms at first, but catarrh and fatigue are clear signs that *some part of the body is vulnerable to disease, if not already in the early stages of disease.*

We find it is necessary to return frequently to the principle that all organs, glands and tissues of the body function as a mutually-dependent

---

[9]***Taber's Cyclopedic Medical Dictionary,*** 13th Ed., F.A. Davis Co., Philadelphia, PA, p. L-46

community, especially when we have to take care of an underactive organ or any disease condition. We have to realize the liver does not break down in isolation from other organs of the body.

What good would it do to treat the liver if the diet remained unchanged and if bowel activity was still sluggish? What profit is there in treating a disease if the cause of the disease is not taken care of? We have to stop and think about these things.

Some years ago, I received an award from a gathering of doctors in San Remo, Italy. Before I spoke to the audience, several speakers had discussed how to take care of certain symptoms of disease. When my turn came, I said, "We have to remember that 99% of the patient is on the other end of the symptoms. It is the patient we have to take care of, not the disease. If we take care of the patient, the disease will take care of itself."

So in taking care of the liver, we have to look for ways to take care of what is causing the problem.

CIRRHOSIS IS NOT INCURABLE

Not long ago, I had a patient with advanced cirrhosis of the liver and a history of alcohol abuse. He had stopped drinking, but had the enlarged abdomen (due to an enlarged liver) that often goes with cirrhosis. In treating him, we saw great changes take place without our doing anything at all to the liver.

First, he changed to a proper eating regimen to give the greatest nutritional support possible to all body systems, taking care of longstanding chemical deficiencies due to heavy consumption of alcohol. Then he went through my 7-day tissue cleansing program, using my special cleansing process to clean out the bowel, as described in my book ***Tissue Cleansing Through Bowel Management***. In a month's time, he lost 28 pounds from the enlarged abdomen. He could hardly believe the improvement. This is a wonderful, almost unbelievable change.

The same thing can be done over a longer period of time through diet and nutrition. By cutting out refined foods, foods with chemical additives, fatty foods, fried foods, all foods cooked in hot oils, wheat, milk, sugar, citrus, iceberg lettuce, alcoholic drinks, cigarettes and all other substances that are worthless or potentially harmful to the body, and by changing to a diet of whole, pure, natural foods, 60% raw and high in natural fiber, we can cleanse and renew the bowel. But it takes as long as a year to do it with foods, perhaps longer in cases of extreme bowel underactivity.

CHLOROPHYLL—NATURE'S WONDERFUL CLEANSER

One of the greatest food substances for cleansing the bowel and other elimination systems, the liver and the blood is chlorophyll, as found in all green vegetables, especially the green leafy vegetables. The problem we find here is that food greens contain less than half of one percent chlorophyll. Alfalfa, from which chlorophyll is commercially extracted, has only 8 or 9 pounds per ton, about 0.2% when extracted, and alfalfa is one of the plants highest in chlorophyll. Commercial liquid chlorophyll often contains only about 1% chlorophyll. Chlorella has over five times more chlorophyll than wheat grass, and over ten times more than barley grass.

Green algae are the highest sources of chlorophyll in the plant world. Of all the green algae studied so far, chlorella is the highest, often ranging from 3-5% chlorophyll.[10]

Chlorella supplements can speed up the rate of cleansing of the bowel, bloodstream and liver by supplying plenty of chlorophyll. In addition, the mysterious Chlorella Growth Factor (CGF) accelerates the healing rate.

DOES ALGAE BENEFIT THE LIVER?

There are many conditions and toxins that contribute to liver necrosis or fatty liver, and one of the most common is malnutrition, especially diets lacking quality protein (specifically the sulfur-containing amino acids). Diabetes can cause one type of fatty liver degeneration, and excessive consumption of refined carbohydrates causes another. Experiments have been done in the Republic of China, Japan and Germany to see what effects chlorella would have in preventing or reversing various liver conditions, and the results are promising and exciting.

One of the first comparative studies of the effects of algae and other foods (skim milk powder and cooked egg white) on the liver were done in the early 1950s at distinguished German universities in Bonn and Cologne. Dr. Hermann Fink fed groups of rats single-food diets to see how algae compared with known food substances. On a diet of only skim milk, most of the rats died of liver necrosis, while one rat on the egg white diet showed signs of necrosis. All rats on the algae diet remained healthy. Dr. Fink concluded that further research should be done to find out if green algae had therapeutic value for the liver.[11]

BENEFITS OF CHLORELLA TO THE LIVER

In 1975 Japanese researchers published an article in the ***Japanese Journal of Nutrition,*** showing that chlorella in the diet lowered both the blood cholesterol and liver cholesterol. There was a definite effect by chlorella on liver function.[12] The question was, how much protection?

Since the 1930s, experiments with ethionine, a chemical toxic to the liver, had been done on laboratory animals, because ethionine caused liver

---

[10]Ei Hayami, *et al.*, "A Comparison of the Chlorophyll Content of Vegetables and Chlorella," ***Hissu amino-san Kenkyu 6*** (1959).

[11]H. and Herold E. Fink, "The Protein Value of Unicellular Green Algae and Their Action in Preventing Liver Necrosis," ***Zeilschrift Physiol, Chem. 305*** (1956), pp. 182-191.

[12]Masuo Okuda, *et al.*, "The Influence of Chlorella on Blood Serum and Liver Cholesterol Levels," ***Japanese Journal of Nutrition 33*** (1975).

malfunctions similar to those caused in humans from malnutrition alcoholism, disturbed sugar storage, interference with protein and fat metabolism, etc. In the 1970s, a group of Chinese scientists at Taipei Medical College and National Taiwan University decided to see if chlorella added to the diet would protect the liver from ethionine damage.

In their first experiments, Wang, Lin and Tung found that feeding chlorella to rats before giving them the ethionine helped protect the liver from damage and produced faster recovery times. Following up on these studies, the Formosan scientists designed another experiment to see how 5% chlorella supplementation of the diet would affect more specific liver functions. Rats fed the chlorella supplement had lower levels of total liver fats, triglycerides and glycogen (stored sugar), and less liver damage, than rats fed the same diet without chlorella, after ethionine was given to both groups. The chlorella-fed rats also recovered more rapidly. Earlier experiments showed that malnutrition caused abnormally high levels of glycogen in the liver and high levels of triglycerides due to liver malfunction. The authors of the study concluded that chlorella protects the liver from damage due to malnutrition or toxins when used at a relatively low level (5%) of supplementation.[13]

Bodies of rats, however, don't work exactly the same as those of human beings. The big question is, can chlorella prevent or reverse liver damage in human beings?

In a later chapter, we present many personal testimonies from those who have used chlorella, but here we will give a few testimonies telling what happened when people with liver troubles used chlorella.

Case 1, 76-year-old male, Ube, Japan. "In 1979, I was hospitalized on account of cirrhosis of the liver and diabetes (for 9 months). After being discharged, I continued to receive treatment. In 1981 I began to take 40 chlorella tablets daily, together with CGF (Chlorella Growth Factor). My physical condition improved day by day. Now I do not tire no matter what work I do."

Case 2, female, Hokkaido, Japan. "Nine years ago I was treated in a hospital for a liver problem and released, but two years after my marriage, the symptoms returned. Four years ago, I began taking CGF liquid and chlorella tablets. At first, symptoms appeared but I was told I need have no fear, so I continued. They cured my liver...and now I rely on this natural food treatment."

Case 3, male, 49 years old. "In 1975, I was diagnosed at the university hospital as having alcoholic cirrhosis...and I was hospitalized. The

---

[13]Leng-Fang Wang, *et al.*, "Protective Effect of Chlorella on the Hepatic Damage Induced by Ethionine in Rats," ***Journal of the Formosan Medical Association,*** Vol. ***78,*** No. ***12,***(December 1979), pp. 1010-1019.

doctor told me there was no medicine that would treat cirrhosis and that I should give up alcohol and treat my condition through diet. After I was discharged...my condition did not improve and I was hospitalized many times in succession. If I didn't drink, my liver function tests would fall, but when I drank, they would rise again. In 1981, my condition became very serious with extremely high liver test readings. I was hospitalized for a month until test readings dropped a little, then released. I began taking 30 chlorella tablets a day along with CGF liquid. For 3 or 4 months, there was little effect, and then my liver function tests stabilized at low-normal levels."

The protein-starved fatty liver can usually be reversed by using one or more of the sulfur-containing amino acids. Toxins such as alcohol or ethionine not only destroy tissue but inhibit the use of certain chemical elements by the tissues. So therefore that tissue repair is handicapped by chemical deficiency.

Chlorella rescues a toxin-laden, fatty, mineral-deficient liver by a combination of methods. First, its chlorophyll cleanses and soothes the irritated tissue in the bowel and builds up the hemoglobin content of the blood. Secondly, chlorella stimulates better bowel function and increased bowel elimination, as noted in Japanese and U.S. medical studies. Better bowel function carries off more cholesterol and fats in the waste, instead of allowing them to be assimilated into the bloodstream where they could become more of a problem. Further, the high DNA/RNA content of chlorella directly stimulates liver tissue repair at the cellular level.

The CGF or Chlorella Growth Factor referred to in the testimonials is a hot water extract of substances from chlorella, which assists in growth and tissue repair as shown by many experiments and hospital studies. At the same time, chlorella supplies a balance of amino acids needed for repair. The amino acids, as found in protein, are the building blocks of tissue growth and repair. I feel that chlorella, with its multiple nutritional advantages, corrects or normalizes imbalances, possibly strengthens the walls of cells in the liver, and accelerates repair and replacement at the level of the cell.

As a consequence of the raising of the functional level of the liver, every organ, gland and tissue of the body benefits.

14. HAVE A (HEALTHY) HEART

The cardiovascular system has, for the past five decades or more, been a subject of great concern to public health officials, doctors and millions of men and women in Western nations where heart disease, stroke and high blood pressure have reached epidemic proportions.

At the same time, dietary changes made by millions of Americans have lowered the death rate due to heart attack and stroke, which is a very hopeful sign. There is persuasive evidence that high blood pressure, high cholesterol and high triglycerides are lowered by regular use of chlorella.

Research in 1981 showed that one in five Americans has high blood pressure, resulting in the loss of 26 million workdays each year. At the top of the list of killer diseases in the United States, heart disease and stroke, cause more deaths each year than all other diseases put together.

WHAT CAN YOU DO ABOUT IT?

Factors increasing the risk of cardiovascular disease are stress, high-fat diet, using too much salt, cigarette smoking, alcohol abuse, and not enough fiber foods in the diet.

You can cut your risk of heart disease by finding ways to relax and lower your stress during the day by eating more chicken and fish and less red meat, by cutting down on salt, or using vegetable seasoning instead, by stopping smoking and limiting drinking, and by increasing your intake of fresh fruits, vegetables and whole grain meals. Cutting down on salt (or sodium) will be easier if you know which salt-loaded foods to avoid, as shown in the following chart.

HIGHEST SODIUM FOODS (mg/100gm)

Food	mg/100gm	Food	mg/100gm
Bacon	1,021	Caviar	2,200
Butter	987	Cheddar cheese	700
Catsup	1,300	Olives	2,400
Bouillon cubes	24,000	Canned sardines	760
Commercial bleu cheese dressing	1,094	Bologna sausage	1,300
		Soy sauce	7,325
Canned soups	(approx) 300-800	Self-rising flour	1,079

My patients at the Ranch have been successful in lowering cholesterol, triglycerides and high blood pressure by taking my 7-day tissue cleansing program, as described in my book ***Tissue Cleansing Through Bowel Management.*** Improvement is often evident in the third or fourth day of the program. Changes in cholesterol and triglycerides are documented by blood tests taken before and after the cleansing program.

Patient, S.B., Female, High Triglycerides

"The first time I took the tissue cleansing program, my laboratory blood test showed a triglyceride reading of 938 (normal is 50-200 mg/dL). In a week's time, it dropped to 253. Nearly three years later, after a year of living under high-stress conditions, my triglycerides shot up to 1403 mg/dL. I went through the tissue cleansing again and the level dropped to 325. I realize there is more work to do, but I am delighted with the rapid drop of triglycerides following the 7-day programs."

Note: The triglyceride count and how they were reduced in this patient in just one week's tissue cleansing treatment.

BEFORE

Triglyceride 50-200 mg / dL	Cholesterol <230 mg / dL *
1403	391

AFTER

Triglyceride 50-200 mg / dL	Cholesterol <230 mg / dL *
325	274

Patient, C.M., Female, High Triglycerides, 80 years old

BEFORE

Triglyceride 50-200 mg/dL	Cholesterol 150-300 mg/dL
2544	633

AFTER

Triglyceride 50-200 mg/dL	Cholesterol 150-300 mg/dL
912	440

Arthritic, bowel disturbances and gas, one movement every 4-5 days.

The pictures show what the before and after triglyceride counts, from medical laboratory tests, were for this patient. The changes were made in one week's tissue cleansing treatments.

THE EFFECT OF CHLORELLA ON HIGH-RISK FACTORS

Laboratory experiments with mice by Japanese researchers showed significant lowering of elevated cholesterol and triglycerides by adding 10% cholesterol to the diet. At a hospital in Fukuoka, Japan, 16 patients with high cholesterol were given five grams of chlorella per day, and no anti-cholesterol drugs or low-fat diets were used. Their blood cholesterol levels in three months were much lower than at the beginning of the test.

Since chlorella stimulates improved bowel activity, cleanses the blood and feeds the friendly flora of the bowel, we might expect to find it has an effect on lowering the blood pressure, and Japanese studies have shown this to be true.

Chlorella is very effective in removing the toxic metal cadmium, which is known to raise the blood pressure. An experiment by researchers at Kanazawa Medical University, using both normal and hypertensive laboratory rats. Blood pressure fell in both groups of the chlorella-fed rats, as compared to those on a normal diet, even though the chlorella-fed rats gained more weight.[14]

The same researchers tested the ability of chlorella to "soften" blood vessels in 10 persons, ages 23 to 4l, over a period of two months, using the pulse wave test. Previous experiments in several countries have shown that the time it takes for a pulse wave to travel along a certain length of blood vessel depends upon the hardness or elasticity of the vessel walls. In hardened arteries, the pulse wave travels much faster than it does in normal arteries. The 10 subjects of the experiment were given 0.5 ounce (liquid) of Chlorella Growth Factor and a quarter of a gram of autoclaved chlorella per day. The pulse wave velocity was measured on each person before the experiment and at the end of the two-month period of its duration. Despite the very low dosage of CGF and chlorella, and the relative youth of the subjects, the pulse wave velocity became slower in 50% of those tested. The research report of this experiment did not say whether any of the persons checked in the study had abnormal pressure or not.

THE VOICE OF EXPERIENCE SPEAKS

The testimony of Saburo Hoshino, a 44-year-old businessman from Tokyo, shows what can happen with larger doses of chlorella.

"Twelve years ago, for the first time in my life, my blood pressure reading was 190/120, and the life insurance company diagnosed my condition as essential hypertension. I was disqualified for insurance.

At the time, I began taking 30 chlorella tablets per day. My condition improved perceptibly in about a month, and after three months, I was able to

---

[14]T. Murakami, *et al.*, "The Influence of Chlorella as a Food Supplement on High Blood Pressure and as a Stroke Preventative for Rats," ***Showa 58-nen Nihon nogita gakkai Koen Yoshi,*** (1983).

maintain normal blood pressure at 140/80 without medication. I lost about 13 pounds. For the past 5 years, I have kept my weight at 125 pounds and my blood pressure at 140/85, and have been able to apply myself energetically to the management of the company."

15. CHLORELLA STRENGTHENS OUR NATURAL DEFENSES

I feel that chlorella's main contribution to the body's natural defense system is its beneficial supportive effects on so many of the organs and systems, especially the immune system and eliminative channels. For many years, I worked to develop *My Health and Harmony Food Regimen* so it would be half building and half eliminative, so it would not only supply all the nutrients and chemical elements needed by the body, but would contribute to the regular and efficient working of the eliminative organs to keep the body free of toxic wastes. With this kind of food regimen, along with appropriate changes in lifestyle, I have seen thousands of patients get out of their illnesses. The fact that chlorella both normalizes underactive elimination and stimulates the building of new tissue, gives me a great deal of confidence in its ability to sustain and support the natural defense system of the body.

WE HAVE TO STOP TEARING DOWN OUR DEFENSES

If we allow our tissues to become burdened with catarrh, metabolic wastes, uneliminated drug residues, unnatural chemical additives from foods, nicotine, chemical spray residues from foods, chemicals from polluted air and treated drinking water and other substances the body is unable to expel, the tissue eventually becomes underactive to the point where it becomes prey to chronic disease.

When we realize that the natural defense system of the body is a system of mutual support among all the organs, glands, tissues and systems of the body, then we understand why our defenses against disease can't be strong unless we stop breaking down the body. This is the very first thing I tell my patients.

We find that the strength of our natural defense system depends on how well we take care of our genetically-inherited weaknesses, maintaining the proper mineral density in the tissues, avoiding toxic buildup in the body and preventing tissue underactivity. These four factors are nearly always linked together. If tissue is underactive, it is usually toxin laden; if it is toxin laden, it is usually deficient, in one or more minerals needed for normal function; if it is mineral deficient, it is usually inherently-weak tissue that has been fed improperly, subjected to excessive stress or overfatigued.

If the body is not strong, the inherently-weak tissues are generally toxin laden because of a toxin-laden bloodstream. If the blood and lymph are not clean, the bowel is not clean and not sufficiently active to carry off wastes as fast as it should.

WE CAN'T NEGLECT ELIMINATION

The four elimination channels are the bowel, the lungs and bronchials, the kidneys and the skin. Their primary function is to carry off food wastes, metabolic wastes and toxic materials that can't be used by the body. The bowel is the key to the whole system. When the bowel is underactive, not only is the blood-stream affected, but the other elimination channels are often overburdened by trying to take care of the overload from the bowel. The average activity level of the four elimination channels determines the level of activity of the lymphatic system.

When the elimination channels are underactive, there is usually too much toxic material circulating in the body for the liver to detoxify, too much for the lymphatic system to carry off, too much to be taken care of by the natural immune system. The body's defenses are overwhelmed. Tissues deficient in materials and burdened with toxic wastes become a breeding ground for germ life and chronic diseases. Individual cells cannot maintain their integrity, and cells can no longer ward off disease-causing factors. This is the beginning of serious trouble for the body.

CHLORELLA PROMOTES BOWEL HEALTH

One of the first things we find out about chlorella is that it stimulates and normalizes an underactive bowel. Dr. Motomichi Kobayashi, director of a hospital in Takamatsu, Japan, prescribes chlorella to all his patients who are troubled with constipation. A U.S. Army medical facility in Colorado found that scenedesmus, an algae similar to chlorella, combined with chlorella fed to volunteers over a period of time, increased the amount of wastes eliminated by the bowel.[15]

Secondly, in 1957, Dr. Takechi and his associates in Japan found out that chlorella promoted rapid growth of lactobacillus, one of the bacteria that promotes colon health. The chlorophyll in chlorella helps keep the bowel clean, while the tough cellulose membrane of chlorella (which is not digested) binds to cadmium, lead and other heavy metals and carries them out of the body. The CGF stimulates repair of tissue damage. To summarize, chlorella restores bowel regularity, normalizes beneficial bowel flora, assists in detoxifying the bowel and stimulates repair of damaged, broken down tissue.

Numerous testimonies from Japan are available, showing how chlorella has taken care of lung and bronchial problems, kidney troubles, bowel problems and skin conditions. Some of these will be presented in a later chapter of this book. The main point is, chlorella improves elimination in all four elimination channels, which is the key to detoxification of the body.

---

[15]Richard C. Powell, *et al.*, "Algae Feeding in Humans," ***Journal of Nutrition* 75** (1961), pp. 7-12.

This allows the rebuilding and rejuvenation of the natural defense system as a whole, and the immune system, in particular.

CHLORELLA PROTECTS THE LIVER

Several experiments have shown that chlorella stimulates a protective effect on the liver, as shown by its resistance to damage by toxins such as ethionine. In one German Study, the liver was protected from the kind of damage caused by malnutrition.[16]

Chlorella lowers blood cholesterol and triglycerides, the levels of which are associated with liver metabolism as well as fat intake.[17]

We can see how the protective and cleansing effects of chlorella on the liver support the natural defenses of the body.

A clean bloodstream, rich in oxygen-bearing red blood cells, is the foundation of a strong defense against disease. Chlorella's cleansing action on the elimination organs and liver helps keep the blood clean. Clean blood efficiently carries off toxic metabolic wastes from the cells and tissues. I believe the buildup of metabolic wastes in underactive body organs and systems is just as dangerous as an exposure to air and water pollution, nutritionally-deficient foods, and exposure to chemicals in the workplace.

BALANCING THE TEETER-TOTTER BLOOD SUGAR PROBLEM

Experiments have shown that chlorella tends to normalize blood sugar in cases of hypoglycemia while numerous personal testimonies show it also helps take care of diabetes.[18]

In hypoglycemia, blood sugar is too low, while in diabetes, blood sugar is too high. Proper levels of blood sugar are necessary for normal brain function, heart function and energy metabolism, all of which are crucial in sustaining good health and preventing disease. The liver and pancreas are involved in the regulation of blood sugar, particularly the Island of Langerhans in the pancreas. So, we find that chlorella supports and balances pancreatic functions as well as the other organs we have discussed.

A large-scale experiment, mentioned earlier, with chlorella was conducted on nearly a thousand Japanese sailors on a training cruise from Japan to Australia and back, over a period of 95 days. Two grams of chlorella per day were given to 458 randomly selected crew members, while 513 others served as a comparison group and did not take the chlorella.

---

[16]H. and E. Herold Fink, "The Protein Value of Unicellular Green Algae and Their Action in Preventing Liver Necrosis," ***Zeitschrift Physiol. chem. 305*** (1956), pp. 182-191.

[17]L. F. Wang, *et al.*, "Effect of Chlorella on the Levels of Glycogen, Triglyceride and Cholesterol in Ethionine-Treated Rats," ***Journal of the Formosan Medical Association,*** Vol ***79,*** No. ***1,*** (Jan. 1980), pp. 1-10.

[18]H. T. Lee, *et al.*, "Hypoglycemic Action of Chlorella," ***Journal of the Formosan Medical Association,*** Vol. ***76,*** No. ***3,*** (March 1977), pp. 272-276.

About 30% fewer cases of colds and flu were experienced by those who took chlorella.[19]

A substance called "chlon A," extracted from the nucleic material of chlorella, stimulates interferon production and helps protect cells against viruses.[20]

Another important aspect of chlorella is evident when we look at hospital cases in which ulcers and wounds that refused to heal were treated with chlorella and CGF. Japanese doctors found that ulcers healed rapidly and that wounds which were unresponsive to various medication and treatments finally healed when the patients took oral doses of chlorella and Chlorella Growth Factor.

Experiments have shown that a substance in CGF stimulates both plant and animal cells to reproduce at a faster rate which stimulates healing. For many years, I have emphasized that only foods can build new tissue, and this is the ultimate secret of true healing.

SUPPORTING THE IMMUNE SYSTEM

Science considers the trillions of white blood cells (leukocytes) and antibodies that circulate in the blood and lymph as the body's main defense system against disease. A protein called interferon protects cells against harmful viruses. Leukocytes of various types not only circulate, but cluster together in lymph nodes and in lymphatic tissue such as the tonsils, spleen and appendix. They line the walls of liver passages, where they are known as Kupffer cells, and portions of the small intestine where they are called Peyer's patches.

The "soldiers" of the immune system are said to patrol the blood and lymph, or stand on guard in the lymph nodes, liver, spleen, small intestine and so forth, destroying harmful bacteria, removing foreign matter and taking old blood cells out of circulation. The great scientist Metchnikoff won a Nobel prize for his discoveries about the immune system in 1908.

Cells and antibodies of the immune system can be destroyed by radiation and chemotherapy. Research has shown a significant loss of white blood cells from sunburn alone, since the white blood cells moving through the skin capillaries are destroyed by the ultraviolet light in sunlight. White blood cells (leukocytes) and antibodies both require a balance of nutrients and high-quality proteins. If we are not eating properly, the immune system is harmed along with other parts of the body.

---

[19]Y. and Tanaka, Kashiwa, "Changes Induced by Chlorella on the Body Weight and Incidents of Colds Among Naval Trainees," ***Midori 1,*** (1970).

[20]Iwao Umezawa, "An Acidic Polysaccharide, Chlon A, from Chlorella Pyrenoidosa," ***Chemotherapy,*** Vol. ***30,*** (1982).

The high beta-carotene content of chlorella helps protect the body from free radicals and reduces oxidation damage. It also helps protect against ultraviolet radiation damage.

CANCER-RELATED RESEARCH

Some of the most recent scientific experiments in Japan and the Republic of China concern the effects of chlorella on the immune system in cases of degenerative disease. Several years ago, Japanese doctors discovered that giving chlorella to cancer patients going through radiation therapy or chemotherapy helped prevent leucopenia, the sudden drop in white blood cell count which usually accompanied those therapies. Leukopenia is characterized by fatigue, low energy and low resistance to infections and catarrhal conditions. Doctors found that if chlorella was given in advance of the treatment, the white blood cell count would not drop as low, and it would bounce up again more quickly than usual.

Research at the Kitazato Institute indicated that chemical substances in chlorella stimulated the production of interferon, a chemical natural to the body which protects cells against viruses and which is believed to slow the growth rate of cancer cells.[21]

At the Biomedical Research Institute of Kyushu University, Chlorella Growth Factor was given to mice that were then injected with cancer cells. The CGF mobilized polymorphonuclear leukocytes to attack the cancer cells, prolonging the lives of the mice as compared to control group mice that had not received CGF. Another experiment showed that taking chlorella orally stimulated the macrophages and T-cells of the immune system, resulting in an anti-tumor effect. Researchers at Kanazawa Medical University in Japan and Taipei Medical University in the Republic of China performed similar experiments and concluded that the anti-tumor effect of chlorella was probably due to the protection or restoration of macrophage activity, which is usually retarded in the body by the time tumors start to grow. Macrophages are large cells of the immune system that literally consume and digest tumor cells, bacteria clumps and other substances that should not be in the body. This information was presented at the Third International Congress of Developmental and Comparative Immunology in Reims, France, in July 1985.[22]

---

[21]I. Umezawa, "An Acidic Polysaccharide, Chlon A, from Chlorella Pyremoidosa, ***Chemotherapy***, Vol. ***30,*** (1982).

[22]N. Yamaguchi, *et al.*, "Immunomodulation by Single Cellular Algae (Chlorella Pyrenoidosa) and Antitumor Activities for Tumor-Bearing Mice," ***Third International Congress of Developmental and Comparative Immunology***, Reims, France, (July 1905).

UNITED STATES CANCER RESEARCH WITH CHLORELLA

Chlorella was given to patients with brain cancer in an experiment at the Medical College of Virginia titled, "Dietary Chlorella Supplementation and Its Effect on the Immune Systems of Patients with Intercranial Malignancies." In this study, 25 people were given 100 chlorella tablets and 150 milliliters of liquid chlorella extract (growth factor) as part of their daily diets. All patients had received other cancer therapy, and some were in good general health while others were very weak and in poor health. Most were on strong medication during the experiment.

During the early stages, some patients experienced gas and other bowel upsets which disappeared as their systems became used to the chlorella. The patients, in general good health, responded better to the chlorella than the other patients. The following testimonials, summarized from an article in a special past issue of ***Health World*** devoted totally to chlorella, show results with some individual patients.

John DeAngelis, diagnosed as having a brain tumor in 1976, was operated on that year but still experienced both grand mal and petite mal seizures. In 1986, he began taking chlorella, and the seizures diminished noticeably to minor seizures in the face.

Russell J. Mann was receiving chemotherapy for a malignant brain tumor and began taking chlorella in 1987. He has not become sick from the chemotherapy. He says, "I think chlorella has had a positive effect, especially on my immune system, and it's now a part of my life."

Christine Armstrong was diagnosed as having a brain tumor in 1986, and started taking chlorella in 1987, after having other therapy. Her CT scan showed no recurrence of the tumor.

Charlene Trevellian was given six months to two years to live after a small brain tumor was found to be blocking spinal fluid and causing a buildup of fluid in the brain. A "shunt" was installed surgically to relieve the fluid pressure, followed by six weeks of radiation. She began taking 15 chlorella tablets twice a day and 30 milliliters of the liquid extract daily in 1988. She experienced more energy, fewer colds and general improvement. She outlived the prediction of an early death (6 months to 2 years), and was still improving at last report.

Not all patients felt that chlorella helped them, but it must be realized that there is a point in degenerative disease where reversal or improvement is no longer possible, no matter what is done.

TESTIMONIALS—PERSONAL RESULTS

I want to say that we have to be very cautious about testimonials, because no two individuals and no two cases of the same disease or condition are truly alike. But, the following testimonials, from Japan, were selected from a great many other available testimonials. What we see here is that many individuals who were not being helped by other treatments were helped by chlorella. I feel that future tests conducted scientifically will confirm these findings from testimonials.

Asthma, male, 3 years old. "My 3-year-old child began to have colds at age one with delayed recovery so that I had to take him to the hospital almost everyday. When he became 2 years old, the hospital doctor diagnosed him as having bronchial asthma and said he would grow out of it. At the beginning of Spring and Fall, however, he experienced violent asthma attacks, tonsillitis and fever, giving me great concern. I began to give my child chlorella and CGF solution daily. In 3 months, he was almost completely free of coughing and wheezing. After 6 months, he no longer had colds or asthma attacks."

Kidney Condition, female, 57. "I developed toxemia during pregnancy, followed by chronic nephritis. My blood pressure began to go up and I developed a heart valve condition as well. I lost weight, having little appetite. At the time I began to take chlorella and CGF liquid. The first night I perspired heavily. Gradually, I improved and began to gain weight. Now I am well enough to do housework and have healed completely from my condition. Even my doctor is surprised by my remarkable recovery."

Liver Condition, 22 years. "In 1983, I was told I had Type-B hepatitis and was hospitalized, but my liver function did not improve. Six months later, my parents came to visit me in the hospital, bringing chlorella tablets and CGF daily. In 3 months, my GOT dropped from 80 to 48 and my GPT fell from 215 to 107. I left the hospital. A medical checkup 7 months later showed that my GOT was 20 and GPT was 30, normal values. I owe a great deal to chlorella."

Hypertension, male, 65 years. "In my 50s I developed hypertension and my blood pressure at that time was 200/115. I tried various drug treatments, but they did not produce satisfactory results. At the age of 59, I began taking chlorella tablets and CGF liquid. Now I am 65 years old. My blood pressure is 130/65, normal level. I no longer have stiff shoulders, headaches or weak digestion. Instead, I am in excellent health, leading a very energetic life."

Diabetes, female, 46. "I developed diabetes in 1972 and was hospitalized, but did not improve. I tried herbal remedies without experiencing improvement. When I heard about chlorella, I began to take 30 tablets and 2 cups of CGF daily. After two months, I felt tired and became constipated but continued to take the chlorella. The constipation soon left, and gradually I began to feel better. Five months later, the doctor told me I could reduce my insulin from two injections a day to one a day. I was overjoyed! My health has continued to improve."

Rheumatism, female, 65. "In 1965, I experienced pain in the joints throughout my body. The doctor diagnosed rheumatism; I was discharged 3 months later. My condition went up and down, but by 1982, the rheumatism became so unbearable that I was again hospitalized. This time I improved and left the hospital again. However, I strained myself and became bedridden. I heard about chlorella in 1984, and began to take both the tablets and CGF daily. Within 3 months, the pain in my joints and muscles was almost gone. The rainy season came and passed, without affecting me unfavorably as it usually did. In another 3 months, I was able to take care of myself without any help, thanks to chlorella."

Previously, I have discussed how the whole body—every organ, gland and tissue—is involved in resistance to disease. I have described how important it is to have a balanced diet of whole, pure, and natural foods and to have active elimination taking place through the bowel, lungs and bronchials, kidneys and skin. I have discussed the importance of chlorella on each of these processes. Also, we need to stop doing those things that break down the natural defenses of the body. This is a remedy with tissue recovery and no undesirable side effects. This is the kind of remedy that should be tried first in all non-emergency cases. Because chlorella works on the whole body, as well as strengthening the immune system directly, it is what I recommend most for building the natural defenses.

There is no magic pill or injection we can take to build up the immune system while toxic materials are circulating freely through the body. Antibiotics may destroy bacteria in the body (good as well as bad), but they do not get rid of the toxic waste and catarrh that the bacteria feeds upon. On the other hand, if we get rid of the wastes, the harmful bacteria and viruses will have nothing to feed on.

The reason I am so interested in chlorella is because it produces a broad array of health-building and toxic-elimination effects, without undesirable side effects. To some extent, it is similar to my bowel cleansing program in its results. Yet, as we have discovered, it also strengthens the natural defense system and the immune system of the body. Keep in mind that chlorella is a food, not a medicine.

Unlike drugs, chlorella works slowly, and its changes seem to be more permanent. This is typical of the healing power of food substances, and when we realize there are no dangerous side effects, we can see how this kind of approach is preferable in many cases. We can also understand that if chlorella is taken regularly, the chances of developing any disease or disturbance are greatly reduced.

16. MY HEALTH AND HARMONY FOOD REGIMEN

We cannot live a good life trying to make up for wrong food habits with the right food supplements. I can tell you, a proper food regimen is one of the greatest factors in restoring health and in preventing disease. Without proper foods, we can't rebuild or rejuvenate tissue, or even maintain healthy tissue in the body. Every diet imbalance creates mineral deficiencies somewhere in the body, and deficiency is the first step on the path to a progressive disease.

What I am presenting in this chapter is a balanced food regimen called *My Health and Harmony Food Program,* a regimen I have developed and used in my sanitarium work for over 50 years, with many thousands of patients. I have seen this program do wonderful things for people who came to the Ranch with many different conditions. I believe in it very much.

Chlorella is a wonderful food supplement, and it will work best and most rapidly if combined with a correctly-balanced and proportioned food regimen. Often, we find that we cannot leave disease symptoms behind unless we stop doing those things which break our bodies down and start doing those things that build it up. Even the best diet in the world cannot keep a man healthy who is constantly breaking down due to poor lifestyle habits. Do yourself a favor: Eat right!

RULES FOR EATING

1. **Do not fry foods or use heated oils in cooking.** Frying lowers nutritional value, destroys lecithin needed to balance fats and make food harder to digest. The temperature at which foods are fried or cooked in oil alters food chemistry which is not a safe practice. One of the greatest contributing factors to cholesterol formation, hardening of the arteries and heart disease is the use of oils and fats in cooking or in foods cooked at temperatures over boiling (100°C.).

2. If not entirely comfortable in mind and body, do not eat. We don't digest food well when we are upset or when we are not comfortable.

3. Do not eat until you have a keen desire for the plainest food. Too often we eat simply because it is mealtime, not because we are hungry.

4. Do not eat beyond your needs.

5. Thoroughly masticate your food. Chewing well increases the efficiency of digestion.

KNOW YOUR FOOD LAWS

Food is for building health. You need to have foods that will meet the needs of a vital active life, and the following laws are designed to do exactly that. These are physical laws to be carried out.

1. Food should be natural, whole and pure.

Reason: The closer food is to its natural, God-created state, the higher its nutritional value. Some foods such as meat, potatoes, yams and grains must be cooked. I'm not telling you to eat banana skins and coconut husks. I'm just giving you a practical guideline.

2. We should have 60% of our foods raw.

Reason: I am not advising a raw diet because I like the taste. I'm saying it is better for us. Raw foods provide more vitamins, minerals, enzymes, fiber and bulk, because they are "live" foods at the peak of nutritional value, if properly selected.

3. We should have 6 vegetables, 2 fruits, 1 starch and 1 protein every single day for proper nutrition consumption.

Reason: Vegetables are high in fiber and minerals. Fruits are high in natural complex sugars and vitamins. Starch is for energy, and protein is for cell repair and rebuilding, especially the brain and nerves.

4. Our foods should be 80% alkaline and 20% acid.

Reason: 80% of the nutrients carried in the blood are alkaline and 20% are acid. To keep the blood the way it should be, 6 vegetables and 2 fruits make up the 80% alkaline foods we need, while 1 protein and 1 starch make up the 20% of acid foods.

5. Variety: Vary proteins, starches, vegetables, ftuits from meal to meal and day to day.

Reason: Every organ in the body needs one chemical element more than others to keep healthy. The thyroid needs iodine, the stomach needs sodium, the blood needs iron and so on. We also need a variety in vitamins. The best way to take care of this is to have variety in our foods.

6. Excess: Eat moderately. Avoid a diet pattern using only a few foods.

Reason: The larger the waistline, the shorter the lifeline. Excess in the diet of only a few foods prevents us from having the variety we need to meet all the nutrient requirements of the body.

7. Combinations: Separate starches and proteins.

Reason: Have proteins and starches at different meals, not because they don't digest well together, but to allow for using more fruits and vegetables each meal. People tend to fill up on protein and starch, they neglect their vegetables.

8. Be careful about your drinking water.

Reason: Most public water systems are now highly chemicalized because ground water sources are increasing polluted. Use reverse osmosis water if you can.

9. Use low-heat waterless cookware; cook with little or no water and don't overcook.

Reason: High heat, boiling in water and exposure to air are the three greatest robbers of nutrients. Low-heat stainless steel pots with lids that form a water seal are the most efficient means of cooking food.

10. If you use meat, poultry and fish, bake, broil, or roast it, and select from this group no more than three times a week.

Reason: Baking, broiling and roasting are more acceptable than frying in terms of preserving more nutritional value and avoiding intake of overheated, concentrated fats. Cook at lower heats for longer times to retain the most nutritional value.

I once thought that wheat and milk were healthy foods and I couldn't understand why my patients were not getting well on them. In 1950, the research of a Dutch doctor, W.H. Dicke, showed that gluten, the protein in wheat, can cause such a severe reaction of the wall in the small bowel that nutrients can't be absorbed through the villi, the tiny finger-like projections that take in the digested food particles. This condition caught my attention because so many of my patients had bowel problems, and I wanted to find out why. Millions of Americans have irritable bowel syndrome, diverticulosis and many other bowel problems.

With regard to milk, intestinal intolerance may be due to a deficiency or absence of lactase, the enzyme needed to digest milk sugar, or to a milk allergy. According to Dr. Jean Monro, intolerance of sugar may be due to insufficient insulin secretion from the Islands of Langerhans of the pancreas. Wheat, milk and sugar cause intolerance in different ways. These causes are well established by researchers. Intolerance of these foods is more common than we think in the United States.

When I put my patients on a noncatarrhal diet (basically a gluten-free, milk-free diet), improvement and recoveries became quicker and more numerous. A patient with a severe case of psoriasis who also developed arthritis and diabetes was greatly helped by this diet. I have had wonderful results through this diet with hundreds of arthritis patients. Many diabetics have been helped to reduce their insulin or stop taking it all together. Dr. R. Shatin of Melbourne, Australia, has suggested that multiple sclerosis may be linked to gluten intolerance, and that poor absorption in the small intestine is sometimes linked to rheumatoid arthritis. Other studies have linked eczema with gluten foods.

I have found that any catarrhal condition, any catarrhal discharge, will generally improve if we cut out wheat, milk and sugar, while using a balanced regimen of whole, pure, natural foods.

When we eat too much of a few foods, we are violating the law of excess, which leads to imbalance in the body and creates an unnatural body. When we feed the cells and tissues 54% wheat and milk, this excess forces a shortage or imbalance of nutrients from other foods we should have been eating. Milk-logged and wheat-logged people produce an excess of catarrh, phlegm and mucus, which, in time, will develop into discharges. These discharges are signs of chemical excess or deficiency, a chemical imbalance in the body. Once we realize we are violating the law of excess, it is important to change to a balanced eating regimen.

Corn, millet and rice can be used as alternatives to wheat in the diet. Buckwheat and wild rice may be tolerated well. Nut and seed milk drinks, soy milk and nut butters can be used as an alternative to milk and milk products. Some people can tolerate yogurt well even when they can't take other milk products. A little maple syrup or honey now and then may substitute for sugar, or we can use fresh or dried fruits as sweeteners for those who have extreme intolerance toward any concentrated sweetener.

Japan Food Research Laboratories

AUTHORIZED BY THE JAPANESE GOVERNMENT

TOKYO HEAD OFFICE : 52-1, MOTOYOYOGI-CHO, SHIBUYA-KU, TOKYO
OSAKA BRANCH : 3-1, TOYOTSU-CHO, SUITA-SHI, OSAKA

ANALYSIS CERTIFICATE

No.OS7070146(1) Date : Aug. 15, 1977

THIS IS TO CERTIFY THAT WE,
the undersigned, Inspector authorized by the Japanese Government, examined the sample submitted by the applicant, and obtained the following results.

Applicant : TAIWAN CHLORELLA MANUFACTURE CO., LTD.
Sample : Chlorella G Powder
Laboratory No. : 1
Received : July 18, 1977
Date of Assay : Aug. 15, 1977

RESULTS

Moisture(Dry 5hrs. at 105°C)	1.3 %
*Protein	62.9 %
Fat(Acid Hydrolysis method)	10.9 %
Fiber	1.0 %
Ash	6.3 %
Nitrogen-Free Extract	17.6 %
Ratio of Digestible Crude Protein by Pepsin	77.1 %
Potassium	927 mg%
Calcium	247 mg%
Magnesium	360 mg%
Iron	195 mg%
Phosphorus	1.41%
Total Carotene	51.7 mg%
**Vitamin A Potency	86,200IU/100g
Vitamin B_1	2.37 mg%
Vitamin B_2	6.15 mg%
Vitamin B_6	0.98 mg%
Total Vitamin C	21.4 mg%
Vitamin E	3.9 mg%
Folic acid	63.3 μg %
Nicotinamide	29.6 mg%
Total Xanthophyll	268 mg%
Total Chlorophyll	2.11 %

Bacterial total count	7.2×10^3 /g
Coliform group	negative
Arginine	3.36 %
Lysine	3.40 %
Histidine	1.11 %
Phenylalanine	2.89 %
Tyrosine	1.92 %
Leucine	4.97 %
Isoleucine	2.49 %
Methionine	0.97 %
Valine	3.46 %
Alanine	4.79 %
Glycine	3.31 %
Proline	2.58 %
Glutamic acid	6.64 %
Serine	2.30 %
Threonine	2.91 %
Aspartic acid	5.18 %
Tryptophane	1.25 %
Cystine	0.63 %

* $N \times 6.25$

** as Carotene $0.6\gamma = 1$ IU

- The end -

Japan Food Research Laboratories

JAPAN FOOD RESEARCH LABORATORIES

Inspector

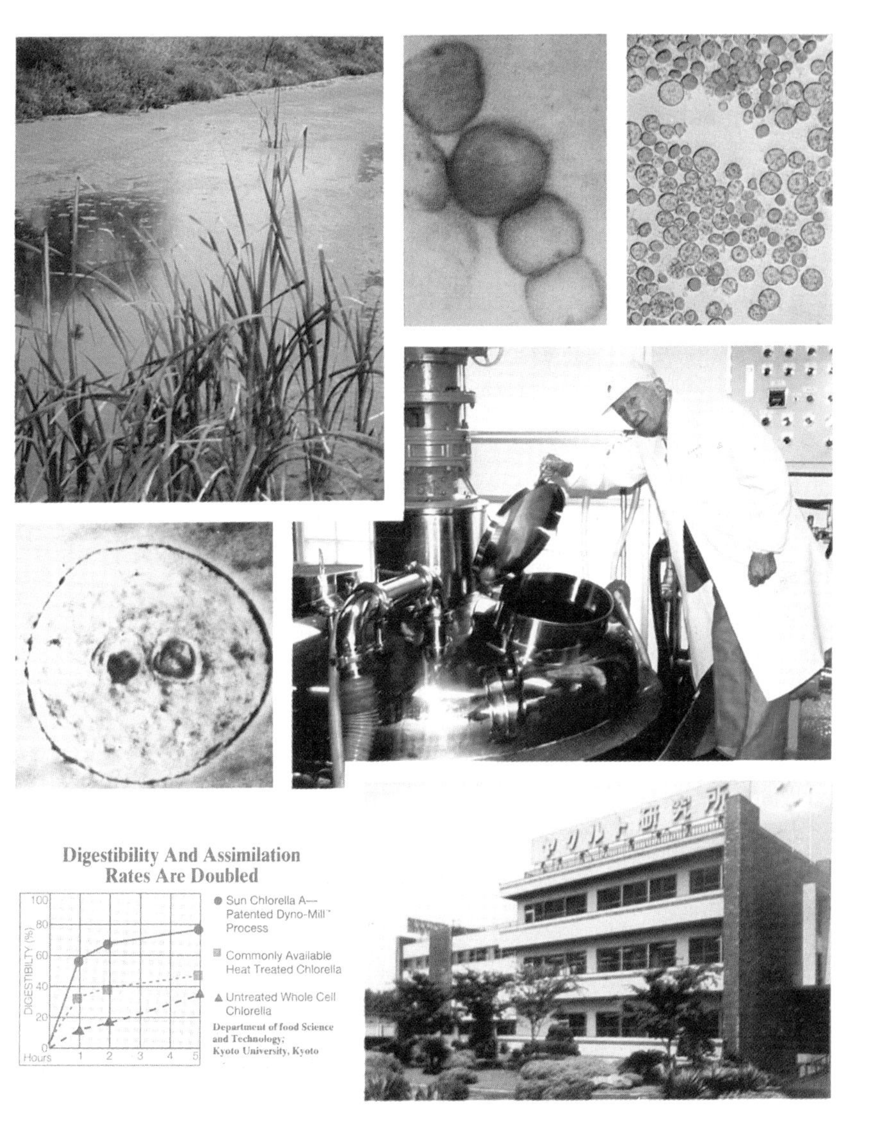

Top Left—Algae grow naturally anywhere in the world where moisture and mineral nutrients are exposed to sunlight. It has taken man's ingenuity, however, to recognize its potential as a food source. **Top Center**—Pre-Cambrian Chlorella fossil. (X3000) **Top Right**—Magnification of Chlorella cell. (X600) **Center Left**—Localization of C.G.F. in chlorella cell. It can be clearly seen that stained C.G.G. are located in nucleus. **Center Right**—Dr. Jensen examines parts of the huge chlorella spray drier at Sun Chlorella Company's factory at Toyama, Japan. **Bottom Left**—Table showing digestibility and assimilation rates of chlorella. **Bottom Right**— Yakult Institute of Japan, which produces a fermented milk-chlorella product with a very high lactobacillus content. Lactobacillus, one of the "friendly" bowel bacteria, is often suppressed by undesirable, putrefactive bowel bacteria if the diet isn't right. Dr. Yoshiro Takechi found that a small amount of chlorella dramatically increased the production rate of lacto-bacillus, so chlorella was added to fermented milk drinks. Chlorella is the best way to improve bowel health. This is why Dr. Jensen has introduced the use of chlorella into his products.

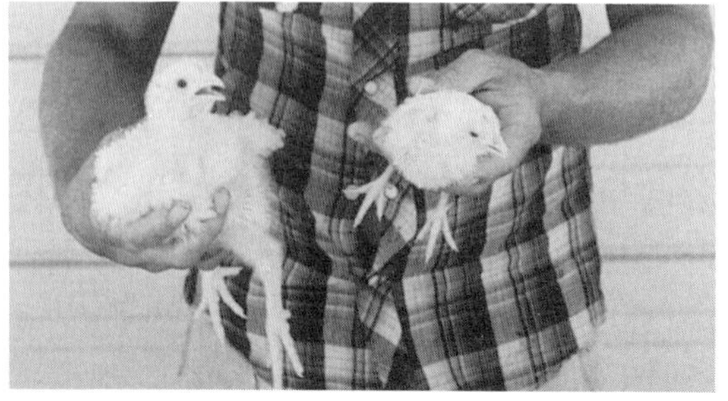

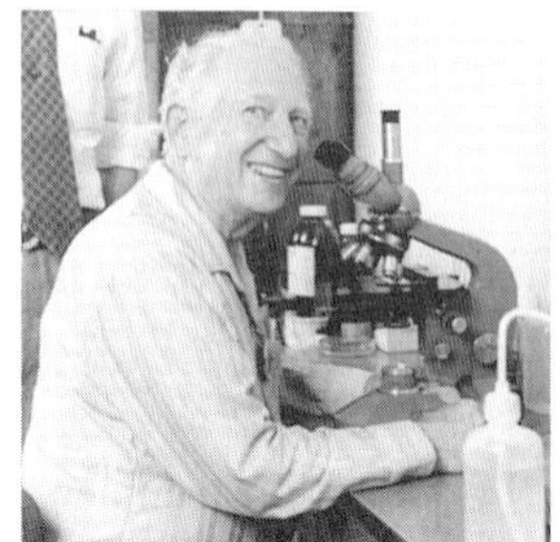

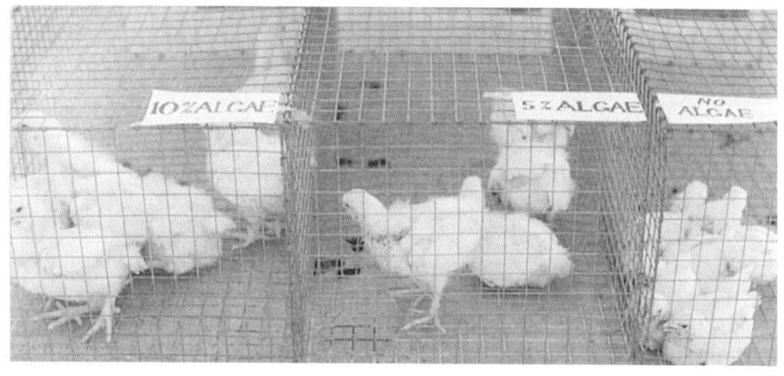

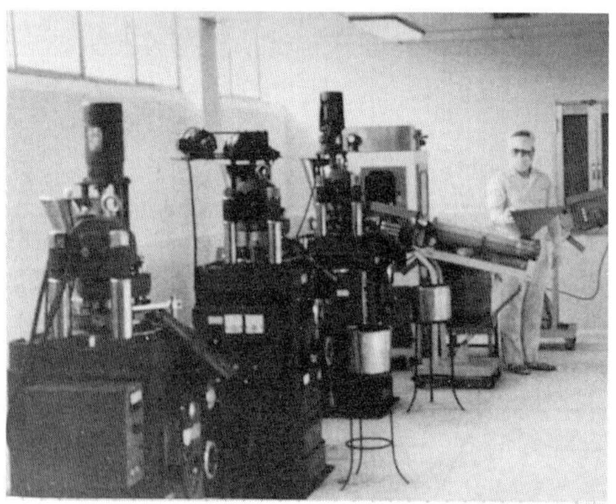

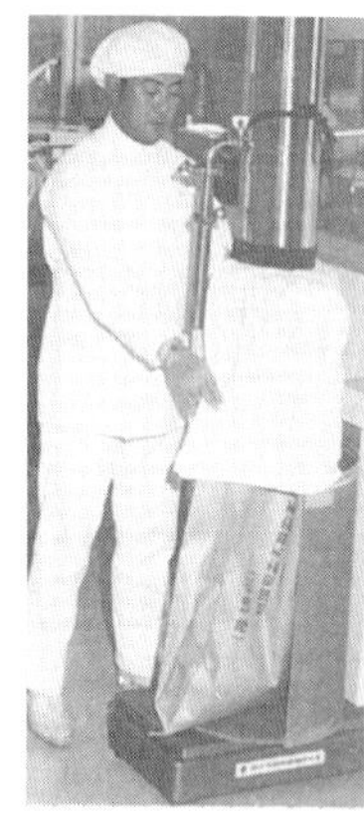

Top Left—Two chicks, same age. Chick on left had 10% chlorella in its feed. Chick on right was given regular chick feed. **Top Right**—I thoroughly enjoyed being a part of the chlorella development process. **Center**—Baby chicks with 10% chlorella in their regular feed outgrew chick fed 5% chlorella. Both outgrew control chicks, given regular feed only. All chicks were hatched at the same time. I saw this experiment myself in the United States. **Bottom Left**—Chlorella is processed under immaculate conditions. **Bottom Right**—Chlorella powder drops from the spray drier into shipping bags and is automatically weighed. Technician seals the bag of chlorella for shipping. Dr. Jensen has introduced this product to a lot of people who have received good results with its use.

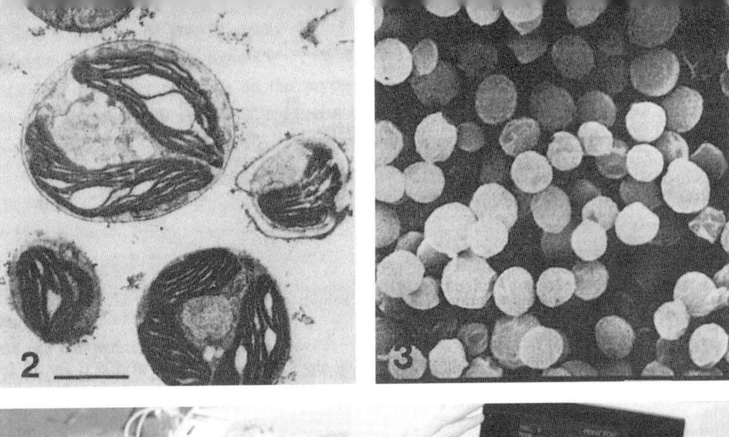

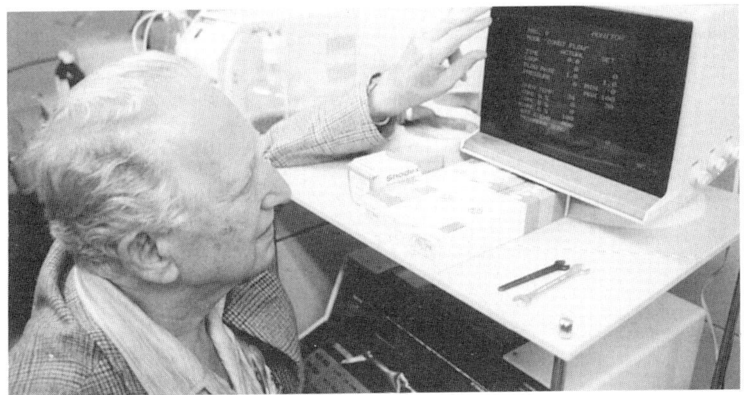

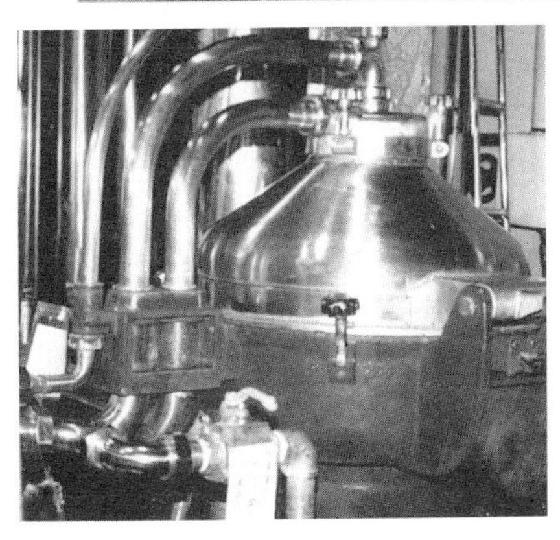

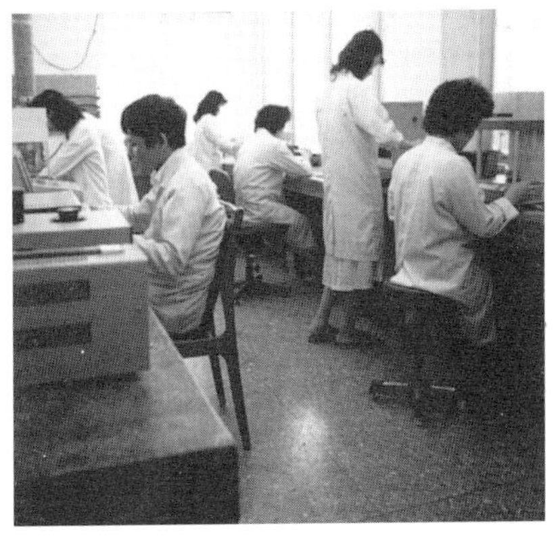

Top—Chlorella pyrenoidosa is the best of the known edible algae. It has maintained a pure genetic structure for 2.5 billion years, as verified by examination of fossil remains of chlorella pyrenoidosa. Its ultra-rapid growth and reproduction rate (quadruples every 20 hours) is due to nucleic characteristics which stimulate tissue repair in humans and hasten recovery from many known ailments. High in chlorophyll, chlorella stimulates blood cleansing and feeds the "friendly" flora of the bowel; chlorella's tough outer cell wall keeps out contaminants until chlorella is harvested and processed to break down the cell wall for better digestibility. Fragments of the cell wall (cellulose) adhere to and remove heavy metals like cadmium, lead and mercury from the body. **Center**—Here I am looking at the computer readout showing the density and retention time of the chlorella in one of the steps of processing. **Bottom Left**—Another example of a chlorella manufacturer proving the extremely clean equipment used in the production. **Bottom Right**—Lab technicians meticulously scrutinize all levels of the chlorella processing. Most tests showing best results in animal and human experiments come from using algae pyrenoidosa.

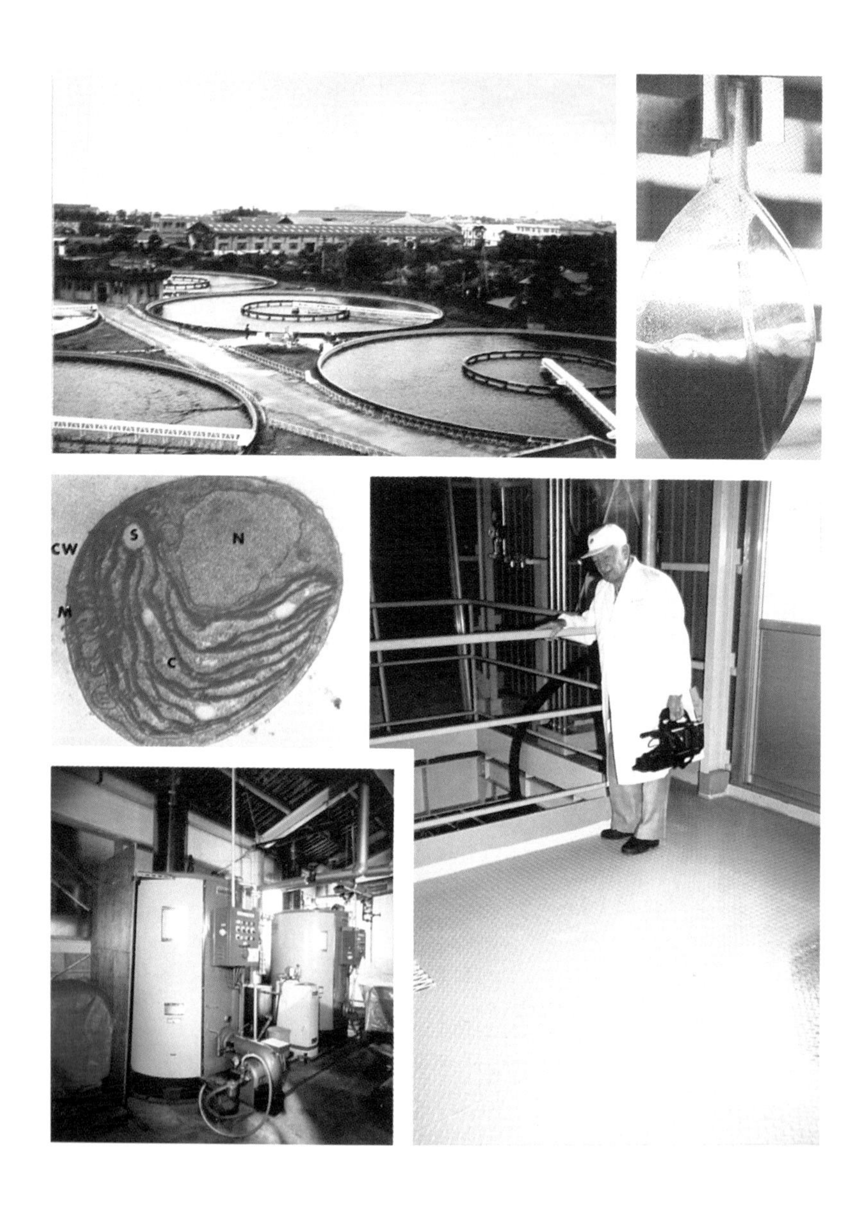

Top Left—These large culture pools are over 175 feet in diameter. When the chlorella in them multiplies to a certain density factor, it is harvested for processing. **Top Right**—The chlorella cells are chemical constituents in the growth medium to make plant food. **Center Left**—Chlorella Pyrenoidosa. Cross section of a chlorella cell at 31,200X magnification under the electron microscope. The cell wall, which protects the chlorella cell from contamination and deterioration is shown as CW. The cell contains a cuplike chloroplast (C) which holds chlorophyll, a nucleus (N), mitochondria (M) which convert food to energy, and starch grains (S). The nucleus is surrounded by a double envelope (NE) with openings called nuclear pores (NP). This is the center for amino acids. **Bottom Left**—Fukuchiyama plant. **Right**—At the Toyama factory. "You could eat off the floor; it was so clean."

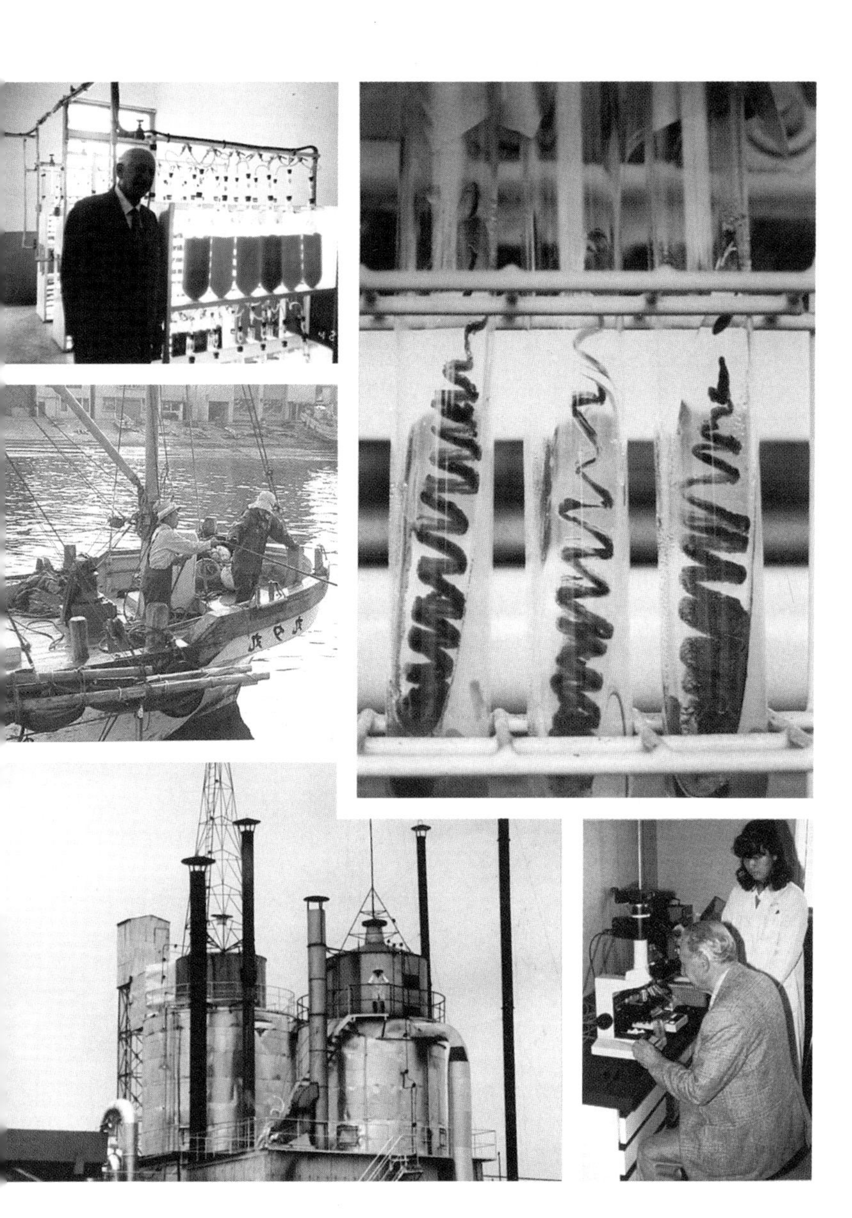

op Left—Culture is put into large flasks for for various stages of growth. Entire rooms are taken ɔ with the developing of seed cultures. **Center Left**—Dietary emphasis on foods from the sea has ɛen linked with the relatively low incidence of heart disease in Japan. **Right**—In the laboratory ᶠ Sun Chlorella's Okinawa plant a close-up of active culture, species selection by agar culture ˌedium. **Bottom Left**—Huge spray driers process chlorella harvested from pools. **Bottom ight**—Analysis room. Here I observed the disintegrated cell-wall chlorella which now has ˌcreased overall digestability to 100%.

Why I Recommend the Use of Chlorella— The Sunlight Essence for Your Health

Chlorella is a whole, pure, natural food, meeting the requirements of the most important of all food laws. I consider it one of the greatest foods I have encountered. I feel that my discovery of the use of chlorella pyrenoidosa and the breaking down of the hard outer shell does more good for the health of all individuals than anything with which I have been involved. I am always open to new ideas to help my own health as well as the health of my patients. I have made a lot of new discoveries over the years in my search for health and the secrets of longevity.

My wife, Marie, and I have been using chlorella since 1983, an we feel it has helped us tremendously in maintaining our good health When asked what I eat and take as supplements, the response is that have been using chlorella. It helps to raise the health level of the patient.

Chlorella is **whole**. It is not subjected to any detrimental refinin process. The whole cell with all the nutrients necessary to support li is available.

It is **pure**. Chlorella is not exposed to chemical pesticides or agricultural chemicals. No preservatives, artificial coloring or flavoring—no chemical additives. It is monitored for purity from beginning to end.

Chlorella is **natural**. It is as nature made it, including the long life and healing factors from the cell nucleus. It changes carbon dioxide into oxygen and waste into a non-pollutant in the body.

It is **digestible**. The cell wall disintegration process has increase digestibility to 80%, which is 20-to-40% higher than chlorella used i the past.

High Chlorophyll. Chlorella content is 2-3% chlorophyll, high than any other known plant source. Chlorella contains 20 times more chlorophyll than alfalfa. Chlorophyll is one of the most effective natural tissue-cleansing agent known.

Nutrients. Protein 55-65%, carbohydrates 20-25%, fats 5-15%. Contains 19 amino acids, including all the essential amino acids needed by the body. Fats are 82% unsaturated, 18% saturated.

Vitamins. Includes Pro-vitamin A, B-1 (thiamine), B-2 (riboflavin), B-3 (niacin), B-6 (pyridoxine), B-12, pantothenic acid, folic acid, biotin, PABA, inositol and vitamin C.

Minerals. Iron, phosphorus, magnesium, calcium, iodine, zinc, potassium, sulfur and trace amounts of manganese, sodium and chlorine.

Bowel Normalization. Chlorella helps restore the underactive bowel to regularity; it cleans and deodorizes the bowel.

Lactobacillus Acidophilus. Chlorella greatly multiplies the friendly bowel flora such as lactobacillus acidophilus and increases levels of the B-vitamins in the bowel.

Bowel Cleansing and Building. The chlorophyll in chlorella helps cleanse the blood while the iron, B-12 and folic acid aid in building new red blood cells.

Heavy Metals. Toxic heavy metals such as mercury, cadmium, lead and arsenic sprays are carried out of the body through the elimination channels by chlorella. Nucleic substances in chlorella activate the immune system macrophage to remove foreign material such as herbicides, pesticides, drugs and free radicals from the blood and lymph.

Liver Protection. Animal experiments show that chlorella helps protect the liver from some toxic materials.

Heart. Research shows that Chlorella Growth Factor in chlorella assists in the prevention of episodes of rapid heartbeat, inhibits irregular heartbeat and reduces heart response to stimuli that normally produce symptoms of over excitement.

Hypertension. High blood pressure is reduced, in many cases, after chlorella has been taken for several months. Blood cholesterol and triglycerides have been known to be lowered.

Growth Factor. Nucleic material of chlorella stimulates cell division, tissue repair and healing, as shown in Japanese hospital reports and studies. Chlorella is 10% RNA and 3% DNA, the long life factor.

Acid/Alkaline Balance. Chlorella neutralizes the excess acids and heavy acidic materials in the body, restoring the acid/alkaline balance.

Immunity. The latest research shows that chlorella activates the immune response and increases levels of B- and T-cells and interferon.

The products I have formulated are specifically designed for the 1990s, with the health problems experienced today caused by environmental pollution, etc. All my products are natural, whole, pure, and they contain chlorella. Chlorella takes care of the whole body, including the bowel, kidneys, lungs. I feel everyone needs chlorella for their health, and that is why I believe in it very much and recommend it to others. For better health you should investigate the available products specifically designed using this algae.

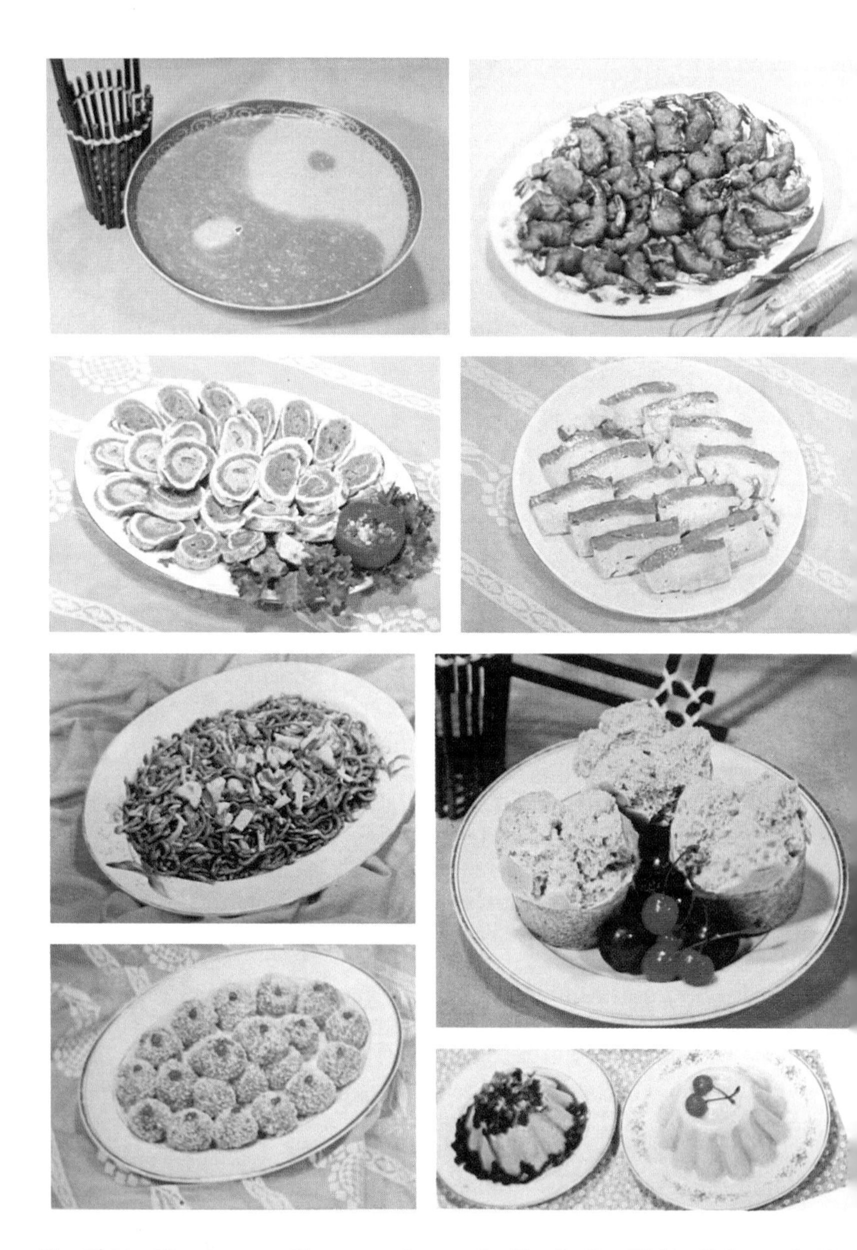

Top Right—Yin-yang soup. The green, of course, is chlorella. **Top Right**—Shrimp cooked in chlorella-laced tempura batter. **Center Top Left**—The Japanese enrich many of their foods wi chlorella, like these colorful hors d'oeuvres. Center Top Right—Slices of tofu with chlorella add to the top layer. **Bottom Center Left**—Fish or shellfish chunks in a bed of chlorella noodle **Bottom Center Right**—Yogurt fortified with chlorella dramatically bolsters the lactobacill content, a wonderful benefit. **Bottom Left**—Raisin-rice cakes with chlorella. **Botto Right**—Dessert ala chlorella. Dietary emphasis on foods from the sea has been linked with th relatively low incidence of heart disease in Japan. Dr. Jensen has recommended ways to u chlorella in many products as well as in his own supplements.

REFERENCES:

Cecil Textbook of Medicine, 17th Edition, Wymgarden and Smith, editors, W.B. Saunders Co.,1985, pp. 727-734.

Gastrointestinal Diseases, 3rd Edition, M.H. Sleisenger and J.S. Fordtran, editors, W.B. Saunders Co., 1983 pp. 1050-1067.

Wheatless Cooking, Lynette Coffey, Greenhouse Publications pty, lt., 385-387 Bridge Road, Richmond, Victoria, Australia, 1984.

Good Food, Gluten Free, Hilda Cherry Hills, Henry Doubleday Research Association, Bocking, Braintree, Essex, England (undated).

"American Journal of Digestive Disorders," article by J.R. Collins, July 1966, p. 564.

Note: For further reading on these topics, I highly recommend my book ***Vibrant Health from Your Kitchen*** for a wealth of nutritional information, and for further details about the effects of using too much milk, wheat and sugar in the diet.

17. WHY I RECOMMEND CHLORELLA

Although a certain amount of mystery surrounds chlorella's role in preserving health and contributing to the reversal of disease, research has uncovered much fascinating information about the health-influencing properties of this potent food supplement.

PUTTING FIRST THINGS FIRST

The most important aspect of chlorella is the presence of a substance called Chlorella Growth Factor (CGF), which can be extracted from chlorella and is now being sold as a separate product. Experiments have shown that it speeds up the growth of children and various types of animals, and increases the rate of healing in the tissue. Chlorella is 3% ribonucleic acid (RNA) and 0.3% deoxyribonucleic acid (DNA), one of the highest nucleic acid contents of any known food substance. RNA and DNA, taken in foods, provide materials for cellular repair and revitalization, contributing to rapid healing, more youthful energy and appearance and longevity. CGF contains a nucleotide-peptide molecule including sulfur and six natural sugars. The peptide segment contains six amino acids, including glutamic acid, which is known to enhance brain activity. In our next chapter entitled, "Does It Work? Yes!," you can see how some very difficult physical problems were taken care of in people who used chlorella and CGF.

Secondly, chlorella contains the highest percentage of chlorophyll in the known plant world, from 1.7% to 7%. The chlorophyll molecule is very similar to the hemoglobin molecule in blood, and it acts as a wonderful cleanser in the bowel, kidneys, liver and bloodstream. Green plants help build red blood cell count and control calcium in the body. Greens help build the number of beneficial bacteria in the bowel and reduce undesirable putrefactive bacteria in the colon. Greens help stimulate bile release from the gallbladder, improving the digestion and assimilation of fats. Chlorella contains as high as 7% chlorophyll, 35 times more than we find in alfalfa. An experiment by the U.S. Army showed that animals fed chlorophyll-rich greens survived twice as long as other animals when all were exposed to fatal levels of radiation. Another experiment by scientists at National Taiwan University showed that chlorella helped protect rats from liver damage when they were fed a toxic chemical named ethionine.

Thirdly, the protein content of chlorella is over 50% by weight, and the digestibility of the best chlorella available is 80%. Cells cannot grow or repair without protein. Analysis of chlorella shows an amino acid balance similar to that of the egg, which is the standard by which other proteins are measured for nutritional value.

Fourthly, the vitamin A in chlorella helps to strengthen the mucous membranes to keep out disease-producing organisms. Other experiments have shown that chlorella strengthens the immune system, eliminates toxic heavy metals such as cadmium from the body, reduces cholesterol levels, stimulates bowel activity and reduces high blood pressure.

When I was in Taiwan, experiments with chlorella showed that this algae has an affinity for heavy metals, and in this industrial age, we find many metals (such as lead, mercury and cadmium) are settling in the tissues so that the need for a cleansing agent which can remove them is very great. In Alzheimer's disease, the amount of aluminum in the brain tissue has been found to be many times normal. Chlorella is one of the best detoxifiers available because of the great amount of chlorophyll it contains.

We have to realize that chlorella is not a panacea, a cure for everything that ails mankind. It is a food, not a medicine. But, if we look at the conditions helped by chlorella, we find that symptoms disappear, not because we are treating a disease, but because we are supplying a high-grade nutrient that cleanses and strengthens the body so it can heal itself. When the cause of the trouble is taken care of, symptoms automatically leave the body without being treated.

When we put together all the previously described characteristics of chlorella, we find that the chlorella strategy is well designed to prevent or reverse many disease processes common in the industrial nations.

In all the experiments on chlorella, you may not find anything mentioned about the lungs. In my work, I have found that if I take care of the patient's bowel, the lungs take care of themselves. Many conditions in the body in various organs are caused by one or more toxic, underactive organs elsewhere in the body. If, through nutrition, we can take care of the main problem, the secondary problems disappear.

Asthma and allergies are helped a great deal by bowel cleansing processes. I have not yet found a patient whose system is allergic to or intolerant of chlorella. In persons with a history of allergy, we find that a rash, pimples, boils or an eczema-like reaction may appear at first as toxic material is expelled from the body.

Those taking chlorella for the first time may experience reaction symptoms as the body gets rid of catarrh and toxic wastes. This simply means the chlorella is working to restore normal chemical balance in the body. Chlorella also takes out bacteria that may be causing problems. Those who need cleansing the most may have the strongest reactions.

We find that the average person does not get enough green vegetables in the diet, and chlorella helps compensate for that. The average person may not have proper bowel elimination, and chlorella helps make up for that. The average woman does not have enough iron or calcium, especially after age 40, and chlorella is high in both. The average person does not repair and rebuild tissue fast enough, and chlorella helps speed it up. These are some of the reasons why chlorella has such a positive effect on health. It is the chemical nature of this algae, a sun plant high in chlorophyll and growth factor, that makes it so active in the body. Chlorella is packed with concentrated sunlight energy, which it is genetically designed to hold; and sunlight is a cleanser. Nutritional factors, such as chlorella, should be considered first in any approach to a chronic disease.

WE MUST TAKE THE HIGHER PATH

One of the hardest lessons to teach those who have come through difficult health problems, in my experience, is that they cannot go back to their old lifestyle without inviting more health problems. Chlorella is an excellent concentrated food supplement, but it can't make up for continued bad health habits. A proper diet and regular exercise are essential for continuing good health.

18. DOES IT WORK? YES!

The first testimonials used here have been translated from the original Japanese language accounts of chlorella users and give some idea of the benefits people have experienced from chlorella. Others have been added from the United States after the Japanese testimonials, but chlorella has not been used in the United States as long as it has in Japan.

No medical claims are being made for chlorella. I know that chlorella is a food, not a medicine. We should realize, however, that when the proper foods are used, together with the right supplements to build up the health level of the body, diseases are often "crowded out." This is nature's way of healing the body.

To put it very simply, there is no room for disease in a healthy body. I feel that nature does the curing, but sometimes it needs an opportunity.

When the tissues are cleansed and strengthened, and when we have removed the obstacles to healing that drag on all the glands and organs, I feel the body heals of its own accord.

Dr. William Albrecht taught that "disease preys on an undernourished body." This is as true for Japan as well as the United States, and I am sure that within a few short years, we will have testimonials about chlorella from people in many countries.

Since chlorella first came out, thousands of persons have been helped by it. The following testimonials have been gathered from Japan over a period of several years, but there are many more than these available.

Very few of the following testimonials mention balancing the diet, and I am certain that if a proper diet was used along with chlorella, results would come faster. I am not making any medical claims for chlorella or CGF (Chlorella Growth Factor), and it is not correct to assume that if someone else's health problem was helped by a certain supplement, it will also help your problem. Still, university studies show chlorella is a very unique substance in stimulating the cleansing and rebuilding of body tissue, and it would be unfair to cast doubt on the testimonials of these people too.

I believe all testimonials should be regarded with caution. Symptoms may disappear for a while without real healing taking place, then return later. However, there are no side effects to chlorella, as there are with drugs. It is likely that tissue repair is taking place, not just symptom relief. Chlorella is a food, and foods are needed for repair, rejuvenation and rebuilding tissue.

So read the following with objectivity and fairness. The chlorella tablets mentioned in the following accounts are 200 mg, while a "cup" of CGF is 30 cc, or a little more than one liquid ounce. The "cup" refers to the cap on the bottle, which is used to measure the amount taken, usually once or twice a day.

The original testimonials have been edited to shorten the length.

Rheumatism. Toshiko Kinoshita (housewife, Uji City). For the last 10 years, I have had severe rheumatism and have suffered from pain in various parts of the body. I tried all kinds of medicine, but none was effective.

By chance, I began to take chlorella. It cleared up my constipation and my bowel movements became regular. After I had taken one cup of CGF and 25 chlorella tablets daily for about a month, the places that had previously been painful began to hurt more and I began to sweat profusely. I heard that this was due to the expulsion of toxins, and I continued the chlorella treatments. As I did so, the reading on the rheumatism test, which had previously been +6, came to be negative. I lost 5 pounds, and my body felt very good.

Rheumatism, Colds. Azuma Ochi (48, Imaji). From my youth, I caught cold very easily and suffered from colds more than half of each year. In addition, I had sore shoulders and headaches frequently. Two or three times a week, I had injections for my shoulders. Then two or three years ago, the fingers of my right hand became painful and changed in appearance. It was diagnosed as rheumatism. I tried various treatments but gradually the fingers of my left hand began to hurt and to change appearance. Neither the expensive Chinese-style medicine nor the heating pad my daughter bought for me had any effect, and I became increasingly discouraged. Half believing and half skeptical, I began to take chlorella. By New Year's my right hand still hurt from time to time, but my left hand was completely free of pain. Now I am 100% cured. This winter I didn't miss a single day of work because of colds and I have stopped taking injections for my shoulder. My four grandchildren all love chlorella.

Rheumatism, Liver Problems. Nae Ikuta (Aichi Prefecture). In June of the year before last, I was diagnosed as having rheumatism of the joints. The doctor told me there was no effective medication for my condition and that a prolonged recuperation would be necessary. From then on, for about a year, I tried all sorts of medicines and substances which were said to be effective but without success. In addition, because I had taken too much medicine, I developed a liver problem, for which I was hospitalized. After this, I heard about chlorella and began taking 30 tablets daily, together with a cup or two of CGF liquid. In six months, the pain began to subside and an examination showed no sign whatsoever of rheumatism.

Malignant Tumor. Hydeto Nakamachi (35, Kushiro). In June of 1972, my nose became very clogged and I developed severe headaches. When I went to Kushiro Hospital for an examination, I was told I appeared to have a malignant tumor and was advised to go to Hokkaido University for a more thorough examination. There I was informed that I did have a malignant tumor and probably wouldn't last beyond December.

I began using chlorella, 50-70 tablets and 2 cups of CGF per day. By October, I felt that I was well enough to go to work. When I went to the hospital, the doctor was very surprised to find me alive. In comparison with the X-ray taken while I had been hospitalized, the new one showed that the tumor had become very small. Since the chief physician's opinion was that I could work if I wanted to, I began working in November. I continue to take chlorella.

Cerebral Thrombosis. Kyuzan Yamamoto (73, Kyoto). In June 1975, I suddenly became blind; I collapsed and was hospi-talized. The diagnosis was cerebral thrombosis. I think my collapse was due to my drinking. However, for some time I have been maintaining a diet of brown rice and vegetables, and for the last few years, I have been a devoted user of chlorella. After 10 days, when the acute symptoms had improved, I stopped taking the hospital's medicine altogether. Instead, I took large doses of chlorella (100 tablets per day) and CGF (2 cups daily). The doctor who diagnosed me had feared that I would remain half paralyzed and was amazed at my fast recovery. My cholesterol level was low, and there was absolutely no abnormality in regard to blood vessels, muscles and internal organs. After about a month, I was discharged from the hospital. Now in good health, I am working together with my younger colleagues.

Weak Stomach, Spastic Bowel, Weak Constitution. Kikuchi Tadashi (64, Sapporo). Over a period of 30 years, I repeatedly suffered either diarrhea or constipation, due to a weak stomach. In addition, my pancreas, liver, kidney and bladder were all poor, and I could not urinate forcefully. Suffering from these various ailments, I used many different types of medicine. I began using chlorella, and about a week later, I vomited, but since I heard that this was a sign that the beneficial effects would soon appear, I continued. About a month later my stomach improved. Now I am able to eat anything. Also, all symptoms have disappeared in regard to my heart, which was supposedly in poor shape. My stomach gas has disappeared also. It is now one year and eight months since I began using chlorella (for seven months together with CGF liquid). Two months ago, I went to the hospital for an examination and there were no problems at all.

Kidney Problems, Nephritis, Hemolytic Streptococci. Ryoichi Nakaoka (47, Muroran). Around June 1944, I came down with acute nephritis, which later changed into chronic nephritis. Around 1958, I developed a low-grade fever and visited a clinic, but there was no improvement. Then in 1962, I went to the general hospital where my illness was diagnosed as hemolytic streptococci infection. I entered and left the hospital no less than 14 times! Those were truly dark days for me. At the beginning of 1977, I began to use chlorella and in about 3 weeks, my unbearable condition began to improve. I became able to drive an automobile. Now I take no internal medicine whatsoever, but feel that I am getting better day by day.

Hematuria, Nephritis. Kumiko Katayama (Sennan). After I had blood in my urine (hematuria) for a period of 10 months, due to nephritis, I learned about chlorella. I started using it immedi-ately, and after 4 or 5 months, my condition improved. I dreaded examinations, however, and so put it off. When I finally made up my mind and went to the hospital, the hematuria turned out to be negative. I felt very happy.

Nephrosis. Naomi Kojima (30, Aomori). Seven years ago, I came down with nephrosis and stayed in the hospital for a total of 24 months. When I was discharged in October 1989, my urinary protein level was still high, so I began taking chlorella. My condition improved, and I didn't need the hospital's medication. Although my health is now good, I intend to continue taking chlorella.

Eczema, Otitis Media, Frequent Colds, Underweight. Chieko Nakayama (18, Kyoto). Perhaps because I was nurtured on formula milk, I suffered severe eczema since infancy. It was diagnosed as "unusual constitution." My growth was slow. I caught cold easily and suffered from wheezing and otitis media as an infant.

My whole family was greatly concerned. After I began taking CGF and chlorella, I caught cold much less easily. After 6 months, not only had my eczema cleared up, but my otitis media improved and I put on weight. My skin, which had been pale and dry, for the first time, took on a glow of health. While I used to be absent from school nearly half the time, I am now attending without missing a day.

Liver Conditions. Cirrhosis of the Liver, Diabetes. Fukumatsu Muraki (76,Ube). In June 1979, I was hospitalized due to cirrhosis of the liver and diabetes. In 1981, I began to take 40 chlorella tablets daily, together with CGF. My physical condition improved day by day. Now I do not tire, no matter what work I do.

Liver Conditions. Cirrhosis of the Liver, Hepatitis. Norikazu Chihara (49). In 1975, I was diagnosed at the university hospital as having alcoholic hepatitis (cirrhosis). At that time, my GOT test was over 900; my GPT was abnormally high, and I was hospitalized. The doctor told me, however, that there was no medicine that would treat cirrhosis and that I should give up alcohol and treat my condition through diet. If I didn't drink, my liver function reading would fall, but when I drank, it would rise again. In addition, blood blisters frequently developed in my mouth. All in all, I was in an extremely painful, unpleasant state.

Then in May 1981, I learned about chlorella. Expecting to be taken in, I nevertheless decided to try it and began taking 30 chlorella tablets and one cup of CGF liquid every day. For the first 3 or 4 months, there was little effect. However, as a result of continuing to use chlorella and CGF, my GOT and GPT levels stabilized at 20 and 13, respectively. In addition, I no longer have blood blisters in my mouth. My general condition has improved to the extent that even if I occasionally have a drink with friends, there is no change in my liver function reading. This is all thanks to chlorella.

Leukopenia. Keiko Suzaki (25, Hamamatsu). My leuckocyte level had dropped to the 2800-3000 range. After taking chlorella for about 6 months, it is now a normal 6800. I don't get fever, and my health has become good.

Gum Infection. Ryosaku Imanishi (49, Kyoto). I was extremely depressed when I learned from the doctor that all my teeth would probably have to be extracted on account of septic fistulae of the gums. I began taking large doses of chlorella, 50 tablets per day, in addition to drinking CGF liquid. After only a month, some effects began to appear and after 2 months, the doctor was astonished at how much my condition had improved. After 3 months, I was completely cured, without losing a single tooth. This was not the only surprising benefit of chlorella. I reduced my weight, about which I had been cautioned by the doctor. I am now 20 pounds slimmer and in good health.

Ulcers. Sajiro Narita (76, Akita). Sometime in August 1979, I developed a pain in the pit of my stomach about an hour after eating. When I went for an examination, I was told it was duodenal ulcers, and was hospitalized for 3 months. In July of the following year, I had another outbreak. I used a combination of hospital medication and chlorella to treat it, and the symptoms discontinued. Presently, I am continuing to use hospital medicine, together with chlorella tablets and CGF liquid. My examination a month and a half ago showed that I was cured. Now, although my health is good, I continue using chlorella.

Liver Conditions, Hepatitis. Kimiko Tashio (Tokyo). In December 1978, at the time of the birth of my third child, I was diagnosed as having hepatitis. Since both mother and child were infected, we were hospitalized. I was discharged after 4 months, but because I could not do my duties as a mother, the baby was sent to a pediatric hospital and months elapsed. Then my other two children began to complain, so I had them examined. Both had come down with hepatitis. Things became difficult after this, and in 1981, both children were hospitalized. They were released 3 months later, but were absent from school 2 days each week, frequently late on the other days and visibly tired. At this point, a friend introduced me to chlorella, and in desperation, we began using it. In just 3 months, the results of the liver function test had declined to 42, to the surprise of our physician. My son, who is in the first year of junior high school, was delighted to be allowed to participate a little in sports that had earlier been forbidden. My daughter, in her first year of high school, is now attending on time every day. As for me, I am able to spend busy days without fatigue. Happiness and harmony has returned to our household.

Liver Conditions, Hemorrhoids. Kumiko Tamba Hokkaido. Nine years ago, I was treated in the hospital for a liver problem, but left the hospital early because I was needed at work. After this, there were no further symptoms and I thought I was cured. However, 2 years after my marriage, the liver symptoms appeared once again. Since I had to help my husband in his work by driving long distances in a truck, I couldn't consider entering the hospital. In addition, I had developed hemorrhoids from the many hours of riding in the truck. At this point, 4 years ago, I began taking CGF liquid and chlorella tablets. They were able to cure my liver in addition to my hemorrhoids.

Diabetes. Gruru Aburada (64, Sakai). At a physical examination at my place of employment, I was diagnosed as having diabetes and I went for an examination at Osaka Adult Disease Center. Since this hospital was for treatment of early stages of diabetes, they first prescribed treatment through diet. Nevertheless, during the 13 years I went there as an outpatient, I continued to take medication. At this point, a friend recommended chlorella to me, and somewhat skeptical, I began using it. During this time, my health took a favorable turn. At my examination after 4 months on chlorella, my blood sugar level was 119 on an empty stomach and 144 two hours later. Shortly after this exam, a favorable trend was clear. I am grateful for the rapid effect of chlorella.

Diabetes. Zenju Nagai (74, Aichi). For 30 years, I suffered from diabetes. Then last March, I learned about chlorella and began to take 30-40 tablets per day, together with 2 cups of CGF liquid. By about the third month, my blood sugar level gradually began to decline and now is 100, compared with 200 which was previously determined. My doctor told me I had made great improvement, and I think I am nearly normal. My general health is also very good.

Colds, Sinusitis, Weak Constitution. Toy Hosoi (61, Osaka). I have been taking chlorella for the past 14 months. From childhood, I had a weak constitution, often caught cold and was anemic. In addition, I underwent many operations for swollen lymph glands under my ears. I suffered greatly for 30 years from sinusitis. When I began to use chlorella, however, I seldom caught cold, my shoulders were no longer sore and my anemic complexion became ruddy with health. I am very grateful for these benefits.

Sciatica. Sueko Yoshida (64, Fukugawa). I had pain resulting from a herniated disc. However, 5 years later, I was hospitalized because of pain in my leg. It was diagnosed as sciatica, and I underwent an operation for it. Then my eyes became bad and I was greatly troubled by cataracts. At this point, I learned of chlorella and I began to take it. In about one year, it reduced the size of my stomach, and my acquaintances remarked that my whole physical appearance had improved. This encouraged me to continue using chlorella, and as I did, my blood pressure stabi-lized, my cataracts did not develop further, my sight improved, my stomach condition improved and the pain in my leg completely disappeared.

TESTIMONIES FROM THE UNITED STATES

The following testimonials were taken from accounts presented in a special past issue of ***Health World*** devoted to chlorella. All of them are from people taking chlorella in the United States.

AIDS. Bert Bloom. "I was diagnosed as HIV positive over three-and-a-half years ago. About two years ago, I started taking chlorella and continue to take 60 tablets a day. Since taking chlorella, I feel great. I have a lot more energy, and my digestion is better. I have only had one cold in two years, whereas before chlorella, I used to get colds about twice a year. During the time I've taken chlorella, my T-cell count has risen from 500 to 750, and it has been as high as 900. My doctor says he doesn't know if the chlorella is helping, but it's definitely not hurting. I only use chlorella and I don't take any other supplements. Of course, I have made some changes in my lifestyle in general. I eat better. I sleep better, and I've been going to the gym. But I believe chlorella has had a very positive effect on my body. I'm basically real healthy and feel great."

Allergies. William Whitaker. "I have been taking chlorella for almost two years. All of my allergies of many years have disappeared, and I am much stronger and can do much more work."

Allergies. Robert Sheldon. "I notice chlorella's effect in subtle ways. When I go to humid climates, I'm less prone to skin rashes. Also, I feel less allergic to cats than I used to be and have less severe attacks of hay fever."

Asthma. Maria Espinal of Brooklyn, New York, developed asthma about two-and-a-half years before she began taking chlorella. After five months taking chlorella, she is much improved and reports that the asthma no longer bothers her.

Arthritis. Angelia Gutierrez had arthritis pain and swelling in her knees and couldn't walk when she began taking chlorella extract and tablets. Her ability to walk was restored.

Arthritis, Colitis. Linda Giles. "My husband and I have been taking chlorella for over a year. My husband had arthritis so bad he was on crutches. I had been suffering from colitis for over 15 years and had very low energy. My husband began taking 15 tablets a day and I began taking 10. We both noticed immediate improvements when we started using chlorella. My husband is now back at work, and my colitis is much better. Plus, both of us have experienced a noticeable increase in energy since taking chlorella."

Body Odor. Carol Andrews. "With chlorella, I've noticed a reduction in my body odor, as well as gas. My skin tone (facial complexion) also seems improved, with fewer blackheads and impurities."

Constipation. Ann Jorgensen. "Chlorella gives me energy in the morning and seems to have a beneficial effect on the elim-inative system. I have less constipation. I am feeling much better emotionally and in good health as well."

Cysts. Marion Priest. "I had fibrous cysts in my breasts and was always feeling tired. My father suggested that I try taking chlorella. I have been taking 15 tablets daily for 18 months and find I now have a great deal more energy. My cysts have completely disappeared."

Digestive Problems, Constipation. Elba Olivares. "My digestive system had been in bad condition and constipation was a frequent problem. Since taking chlorella, I have noticed a great change in my condition. My constipation is relieved and my digestion has improved dramatically."

Drug Addiction—Cocaine. Mr. A. had previously been unable to kick the cocaine habit because of difficulty with with-drawal symptoms. After taking 2 or 3 tablets of chlorella per day, withdrawal symptoms were no longer experienced.

Eczema. Maria Chrisidis. "I used to have skin eczema. It would occur as water-filled blisters on my hands and left foot. The blisters used to itch and break open into sores. After one week on chlorella, my eczema started to heal. After two weeks, the eczema was completely gone. I continue to take chlorella because I don't want to have eczema anymore."

Epileptic Seizures. Betty Cox. "I have a 17-year-old son, Alex, who started having epileptic seizures about a year-and-a-half ago. The seizures were getting more frequent, about once every two months. Alex began taking chlorella in June 1988, and has not had any more seizures since September 1988."

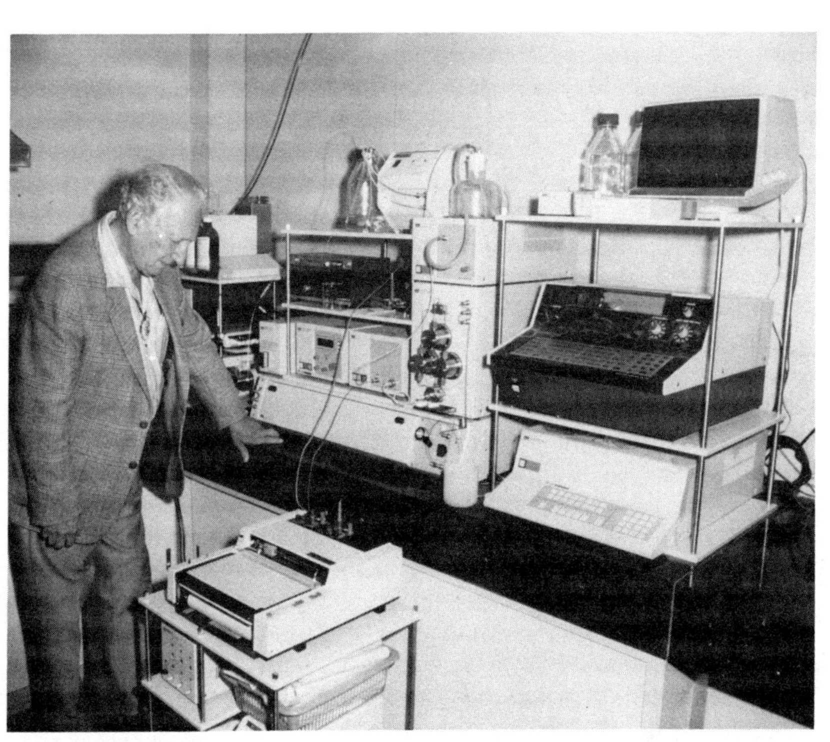

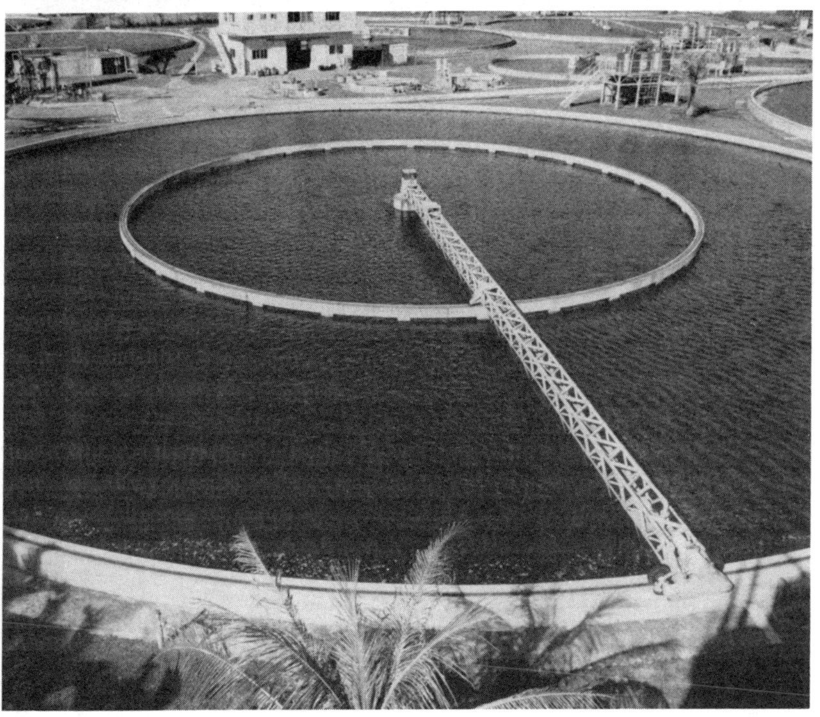

Gout. Theodore Akiba. "I had a painful gout condition in my right foot. A friend of mine suggested that I try chlorella. I have been taking chlorella for about a year and my gout is completely gone."

Herpes Simplex. Teresa Grande. "In July, 1988, signs of herpes simplex were developing on my hand. This had been recurring at intervals for at least 20 years. I started taking chlorella and within a few days the infection disappeared."

Side Effects of Chemotherapy. Marilyn Mosher was undergoing chemotherapy for breast cancer when she began taking 4 to 6 chlorella tablets daily, later increased to 2 granule packets (equal to 30 tablets) daily. Many of the side effects of the chemo-therapy disappeared. Her attitude and energy improved.

Ulcer. Lewis Klein. "I had an ulcer that bothered me for over 20 years. I read about chlorella in a health magazine and decided to try it. That was in the summer of 1987. By October 1987, my ulcer was gone, and it hasn't bothered me since."

These fascinating reports show that chlorella really works, to help rebalance the body chemistry and repair damaged tissue. That is why I believe in using chlorella and advise my patients to use it.

19. WHAT RESEARCH REVEALS

Chlorella is possibly the most thoroughly researched food of our time, with thousands of research papers, from many universities and medical schools published in the scientific journals. Previous chapters, show the great variety of beneficial health effects chlorella has on the human body. This underlines its general importance, but I believe that some readers will appreciate a somewhat more technical discussion.

IMMUNOLOGICAL EFFECTS AND TUMOR RESISTANCE

Four types of chlorella derivatives: 1) living cells, 2) high-pressure-steam-processed agents, 3) cellular wall agents, and 4) hydrothermal extracted agents (Chlorella Growth Factor—CGF) were taken from a pure culture of chlorella pyrenoidosa for use in this experiment. The CGF was further divided into a protein-rich fraction (CGF-prf) and protein-free fraction (CGF-pff).

The findings suggest that high-pressure-processed chlorella cells and CGF-prf activate both groups of antibody-producing cells, B-cells and T-cells. When T-independent antigen (LPS) was used, only B-cells were activated. When T-dependent antigen (SRBC) was used, both B-cells and T-cells were activated.

A second similar experiment was carried out to test the effects of chlorella on mice with mouse breast cancer cells (MMa) and mouse hepatoma cells (MH134). Ehrlich tumor cells were successively cultured in ddY mice. Eight mice out of ten pretreated with autoclaved chlorella survived MM2 transplantation over 60 days. Mean survival time of control group mice was 2l days. No remarkable difference between controls and other groups was observed. The 8 surviving mice were rechallenged with MM2 and MH134. All mice survived MM2, but all rechallenged with MH134 died. Tumor growth of Ehrlich cells was inhibited by about 50% as compared with controls. ("Effect of Various Products Derived from Chlorella Pyrenoidosa Cells on Defense Mechanism of Mice," T. Murayama, *et al.*, Laboratory of Serology, Kanazawa Medical University 1985). A paper on this experiment was presented at the Third International Congress of Developmental and Comparative Immunology in Reims, France (July 7-13), 1985.

INTERFERON STIMULATION

When the acidic polysaccharide Chlon A, purified from hot-water extract of chlorella pyrenoidosa, was given to mice, a relatively high titer of interferon was found in the serum 2.5 hours after injection. Protective activity of Chlon A was challenged by influenza virus and results showed increased survival over controls. Chlon A also showed antitumor activity against Ehrlich ascites carcinoma inoculated into ddY mice (An Acidic Polysaccharide, Chlon A, from ***Chlorella Pyrenoidosa, I. Umeszwa, et al., Chemotherapy, 30 [9]***, 1982).

PROSTAGLANDIN E3

The halophilic algae chlorella minutissima is reported as a source of the rare fatty acid eicosapentaenoic acid (EPA), used by pharmaceutical companies for enzymatic conversion to prostag-landin E3. Under continuous nutrient feeding in mixotrophic growth, mass culture methods were successfully applied to chlorella minutissima to obtain high yields. This species of chlorella was originally found in the ocean around Greenland. Controlled growth methods produced yields of chlorella minu-tissima with 30% content of fatty acids: EPA was 35% to 40% of total fatty acids ("The Mass Culture of Chlorella Minutissima for a Rare Biochemical," S.W. Huang and L.P. Lin, National Taiwan University, Taipei, R.O.C.).

CHOLESTEROL AND TRIGLYCERIDE LEVELS

Male mice of the dd strain were fed a hypercholesterolemic diet containing 2% cholesterol for 7 days, resulting in significant elevation of total liver lipids and cholesterol. The addition of 10% dried chlorella powder to the diet greatly depressed these elevations. At Wakahisa Hospital of Fukuoka, Japan, 16 in patients with hypercholesterolemia were near normal. ("The Effects of Chlorella on the Levels of Cholesterol in Serum and Liver," M. Okuda, T. Hasegawa, M. Sonoda, T. Okabe and Y. Tanaka, ***Japanese Journal of Nutrition, 33 [1]***:3-8, 1975.)

HEPATIC PROTECTION

Researchers in the respective departments of biochemistry at Taipei Medical College and the College of Medicine, National Taiwan University,

Republic of China, studied the effects of chlorella on the levels of glycogen, triglyceride and cholesterol in rats with and without administration of ethionine. Rats with chlorella-supplemented diets had lower levels of total hepatic lipids, triglycerides and glycogen, and showed a less severe reaction to the ethionine than basal diet groups. Chlorella-fed rats recovered rapidly from hepatic injury. ("Effects of Chlorella on the Levels of Glycogen, Triglyceride and Cholesterol in Ethionine-Treated Rats," L. Wang. J. Lin and Y. Tung, ***Journal of the Formosan Medical Association, 79:***1-10, 1980.)

CATARACTS AND LENS OPACITY

Abnormal accumulation of calcium ions in the lens has been correlated with lens opacity and cataract formation in animals and humans. A study of calcium-pump activity in mouse lens homo-genate was carried out by the department of biophysical chemistry, Meijo University, Nagoya, Japan.

The calcium ion gradient across the lens boundary was found to depend, in part, on the activity of Ca-ATPase in the lens. Ca-ATPase, in turn, was found to be activated by calmodulin, a protein which binds to calcium ions in the lens. Calmodulin derived from chlorella was compared with calmodulin derived from bovine brain and bovine lens, and was discovered to activate Ca-ATPase as effectively as the animal derivatives. When calmodulin inhibitors were administered, opacity of the lens rapidly developed. Transparency of the lens may be dependent upon sufficient calmodulin to activate Ca-ATPase and continuously maintain the proper calcium ion gradient across the lens boundary. (Calcium-Pump and Its Modulator in the Lens: A Review, S. Iwata, ***Current Eye Research, 4 [3]:***229-305, 1985.)

HYPERTENSION

At the Food Research Institute at Kinki University, Japan, chlorella was tested to determine its effect on spontaneous hypertensive rats liable to develop apoplexy. Male SHRSP rats, 5 weeks old, were used in both the control group (14) and experimental group (11). Controls were provided standard commercial feed, while the experimental rats were given free access to food and water. Body weight and blood pressure were recorded weekly. Rats which died during the experiment were autopsied. Some were tested to determine elastin content of the aorta and plasma renin activity.

Results: after 7 weeks, experimental rats averaged 20-30 mm Hg lower in BP than controls. Of the controls, 5 died by 30 weeks, 4 revealing cerebral lesions. There were no deaths in the chlorella-fed group during the 30-week duration of the experiment. Renin activity in rats sacrificed at 25 weeks was 16.31+, 8.90 for controls. ("The Influence of Chlorella as a Food Supplement on High Blood Pressure and as a Stroke Preventative for Rats," T. MuraKami, ***Showa 58-nen Nihon nogika gakkai Koen Yoshi,*** 1983.) (See also "Isolation and Identification of Hypotensive Substances in

Chlorella Extract," T. Murakami, Y. Lizuka, Y. Matsubara, K. Yokoi, S. Donda. Kakehi, K. Okamoto and H. Myyake, ***Medical Journal of Kinki University, 5 [3]***:119-130, 1989.)

BLOOD SUGAR LEVEL

Normal male rats, 180-200 grams, were divided into experi-mentals and controls. Experimentals were given chicken chow with 3% chlorella powder, while controls were given chicken chow only. Blood sugar of the chlorella-supplemented rats remained at from 68% to 91% that of controls. ("Hypoglycemic Action of Chlorella," H. Lee, J. Lai and Y. Tung, ***Journals of the Formosan Medical Association, [76]*** *3*:272-276, March 1977.)

SAFETY OF CHLORELLA

In a study of the potential acute oral toxicity of green and yellow chlorella powders, the Huntingdon Research Center, Huntingdon, England, tested groups of rats of the CFY strain by giving them dosages of chlorella powder in distilled water for a 14-day observation period. The LD-50 was found to be in excess of 16 grams/kg body weight. All rats survived the observation period, body weight changes were similar to those of controls, and detailed microscopic examination did not reveal any changes that could be attributed to treatment with chlorella. During the 14-day observation period, no adverse reactions to chlorella ingestion were found. ("Acute Oral Toxicity to Rats of Green Chlorella and Yellow Chlorella Powders," Unpublished report, Huntingdon Research Center, Huntingdon, England, No. 1972).

REGULATION OF HEARTBEAT

Scientists at Kanazawa Medical College in Japan studied the effect of CGF (Chlorella Growth Factor) on the sinoauricular nodes of rabbit hearts. The sinoauricular nodes were cut into smaller pieces (0.5 x 0.5m), and true pacemaker cells were selected from them, cells with an active potential of around 70 mV. CGF addition had the effect of reducing spontaneous discharge, showing a bradycardia effect on heart pacemaker cells. The bradycardia effect inhibited the rising speed of Phase IV, raising the threshold for excitement, prolonging the refractory period, possibly leading to an anti-arrhythmic effect. In a second experiment, arrhythmias were inhibited 1 minute after addition of CGF. CGF may prevent paroxysmal tachycardia, induce steady heartbeats, and alleviate excitability of the myocardium to stimulus. ("Bradycardia Effect of CGF," S. Goto, *et al.*, Second Department of Physiology, Kanazawa Medical College, Japan.)

20. CHLORELLA EXPERIMENTS— A REAL EYE OPENER

Long before the discovery of healing properties in chlorella, feeding experiments were done with various animals to find out if there were any toxic effects in chlorella and whether the protein and other nutrients could be used as foods on their own or whether they would have to be mixed with other foods. The first animal experiments by the Carnegie Institute proved to be very disappointing. Animals fed with chlorella didn't do as well as animals given powdered milk.[23] Experiments in Germany, however, showed the opposite.

Dr. Hermann Fink's experiments feeding laboratory rats with scenedesmus, an alga similar to chlorella, showed such surprising results that he recommended further tests to find out if the alga had protective or healing properties. In his experiments at the Universities of Cologne and Bonn, Dr. Fink found out that the average weight gain of alga-fed rats was 26% higher than that of milk-fed rats after 120 days, and 39% higher than rats fed cooked egg white. Moreover, none of the rats fed the alga diet had liver damage, while many of the milk-fed or egg-fed rats showed severe liver damage.[24]

In Japan, Dr.Takechi made another great discovery. Lactobacillus, one of the "good" bacteria in the human colon, increased fourfold in a standard growth medium after one-half-to-one percent of chlorella was added.[25]

It was about this time that researchers began to assume that chlorella had something that other foods didn't have. Earlier effects on animals' growth were only considered proof of the high quality of alga protein, even though the results were puzzling in some cases. Studies soon showed the weight gain was not due to the high-quality protein in the chlorella.

Arakawa and Kamitachi, in separate experiments using baby mice and rats, respectively, found that the smaller percentages of chlorella added to the diet produced better weight gain than either the standard diet alone or the standard diet with 50% or more chlorella added.

Young rabbits fed soybean flour with 5% chlorella added gained 47% more weight than rabbits fed on soybean flour alone over a period of 49 days. The weights of the soybean group increased by an average of 234 grams while the chlorella-soybean group increased an average of 345 grams.

In another experiment, young pigs ranging from 31 to 44 pounds were divided into two groups. The control group was given regular feed, the other was given the same feed plus 3% chlorella. After 140 days, the controls

---

[23]A. W. Fisher, Jr. and John S. Burlew, "Nutritional Value of Microscopic Algae," ***Algae Culture*** edited by John S. Burlew, Carnegie Institution, Washington, DC (1953), pp. 306-309.

[24]H. and Harold E. Fink, "The Protein Value of Unicellular Green Algae and Their Action in Preventing Liver Necrosis, "***Zeitsch. Physiol. Chem., 305:***182-191, 1956.

[25]Yoshiro, Takechi "Regarding the Growth Accelerating Substances in Chlorella," ***Hissu. amino-san Kenkyu 8,*** 1962.

gained an average of 194 pounds while the chlorella group gained an average of 228 pounds, a 17% gain over the controls. The weight of the food given to each pig in both groups was the same. Other experiments with pigs in which the basic diet was varied, excepting for a small percentage of added chlorella, showed consistent higher percentage weight gains in the chlorella-fed group over the pigs on the non-chlorella diet.

Chlorella experiments with chickens were divided into two parts. In one part, the effect of chlorella on egg laying was investigated, and in the other part, the effect on weight gain of baby chicks was studied. The first experiment, performed by Arakawa, showed no significant difference in the number of eggs laid by the two groups. However, only 13 chickens were used in the experiment. A follow-up study by Nakamura had the same problem—only 14 chickens (Plymouth Rocks) were used, 7 in each group. Four of the controls died before the 9th week of the experiments, so the comparison was made only over the first 8 weeks. The control chickens averaged 0.23 eggs per day (less than 1 every 4 days), while the chlorella group laid over twice as many eggs as the controls. Anyone who knows laying chickens well would say that neither group did very well. Another experiment by Nakamura showed that chlorella-fed chickens started laying two weeks earlier than controls, but he didn't comment on the number of eggs laid. Using 25 chickens in each of two groups, Nakamura's next experiment resulted in an average of 0.52 eggs per day for controls and 0.70 eggs per day for the chlorella group over a period of 180 days. Both groups had standard feed, with 2% chlorella added to the feed of the chlorella group. This experiment indicated 35% higher egg production in the chlorella group. The average weight of the chickens over the feeding period was not significantly different.

Using broilers, Nakamura and his associates performed an experiment specifically to check weight gain, not eggs. Three-day-old chicks were fed a basic feed diet with either 5% added fat or 2% added chlorella for 60 days. Both male and female chickens fed chlorella gained significantly more weight than controls. Chlorella-fed females gained an average of 6% more weight than controls. Chlorella-fed females gained an average 6% more weight than females with regular feed in one experiment, and 14% more in another. (The first group was fed in summer, the latter in winter.) Males fed regular feed plus 5% fat and 2% chlorella gained 9% more weight than males given feed plus 5% fat. A third comparison using all male chicks compared birds fed a standard feed with others given standard feed plus 5% fat and still others with standard feed plus 5% fat and 2% chlorella. The fat chickens gained an average of 1.6% more than the controls; the chlorella-plus-fat group gained an average of 20.6% more than the controls. (After 60 days, the lowest weight was an average of 1.7 pounds for hens fed standard feed in summer, while the highest weight was an average of 2.6 pounds for roosters fed standard feed plus 5% fat and 2% chlorella in summer.)

Regardless of season, chlorella-fed chickens gained more weight and faster than of the others.

I have personally seen the results of similar animal experiments in the United States, and I know these reports are accurate and reliable.

Japanese doctors soon became interested in chlorella. They understood that any food which produced significant weight gains in animals, when used as a small percentage of the normal diet, had something very special about it. But, before we get into the healing work, there is one more experiment—this time with people—which showed that the remarkable properties of chlorella applied equally to humans as to animals.

Dr. Yoshio Yamagishi and associates were given permission to test chlorella on healthy 10-year-old fifth-grade students at Okuno Primary School in Tokyo, Japan. The test group to receive chlorella consisted of 22 boys and 18 girls, while a control group of 22 boys and 15 girls served as a comparison. Two grams of chlorella tablets per day were given to the test group, except on Sundays and holidays, a total of 112 days. Height and weight of all children were recorded on the 2lst day of each month. After the 112-day experiment, the average height increase for the chlorella boys was 1 inch, the control boys 0.6 inch, with respective weight increases of 2.3 pounds versus 1.6 pound. The girls in both groups grew 0.9 inch in height, but the chlorella girls gained an average of 4.2 pounds while the control girls gained 2.7 pounds. This is quite a difference, considering that the only change in these childrens' lives was the consumption of 2 grams of chlorella per day by one of the two groups.[26]

I want to make it clear that *Chlorella is not known to stimulate weight gain in adults, nor is it known to increase the spread of growth rate of any disease.* It only stimulates growth in children and animals that haven't reached their full, adult size. This is one of the greatest differences between chlorella and other foods. Nucleic substance in chlorella stimulates the immune system to act against tumors of some types.

EARLY HOSPITAL TESTS OF CHLORELLA

At the Saito Hospital in Fukuoa, Japan, doctors tried chlorella tablets on stomach and duodenal ulcer patients were not healing. In most, the pain disappeared within 20 days of taking 3 grams per day of chlorella. Other symptoms disappeared in from 2l to 40 days. A miniature medical camera confirmed that new tissue had closed up the ulcers.[27]

---

[26]Yoshio Yamada, *et al.*, "School Childrens' Growth and the Value of Chlorella," ***Nihon iji shimpo***, No. ***2196***, 1966.

[27]Yoshio Yomada, "The Treatment of Peptic Ulcers by Chlorella," ***Nihon iji shimpo***, No. ***1997***, 1962.

EFFECT OF CHLORELLA TABLETS ON THE SYMPTOMS OF GASTRIC ULCERS, PEPTIC ULCERS AND CHRONIC GASTRITIS

Subjective

Symptom	Cases	Cured	Improved	Efficiency
Gastric ulcer	6	6	0	100%
Peptic ulcer	9	7	2	71%
Chronic gastritis	2	-	-	-
TOTAL	17	2	0	100%

EFFECT OF CHLORELLA TABLETS ON THE SYMPTOMS OF GASTRIC ULCERS, PEPTIC ULCERS AND CHRONIC GASTRITIS

Objective

Symptom	Cases	Cured	Improved	Efficiency
Gastric ulcer	6	6	0	100%
Peptic ulcer	9	7	2	71%
Chronic gastritis	2	-	-	-
TOTAL	17	2	0	100%

At another hospital, chlorella and liquid CGF were given to patients with long-standing wounds that refused to heal after the standard medications and treatments. New tissue began to appear in a matter of days, and all of them were soon healed completely. These cases showed that when the body's healing resources were exhausted, chlorella—or some substance in CGF—was capable of stimulating tissue repair.

The ulcer cases and the cases of hard-to-heal wounds are mentioned here because neither the patient's diets nor medication can be given credit for the healing, and because visible evidence of new tissue growth was evident in th cases. Many other diseases and conditions have disappeared after chlorella w taken, but these are sufficient to show that something in chlorella promotes tissue repair.

The original discovery of Chlorella Growth Factor was made by D. Fujimaki of the People's Scientific Research Center in Tokyo, Japan. He fou that hot water dissolved some substances from chlorella which produced wei gain in animals similar to the results obtained by giving them chlorella powder.[28]

The solution extracted from chlorella was not a simple one, but a mixtu of all water-soluble substances in the alga—amino acids, vitamins, sugars, peptides and nucleic substances.

The structure of the growth-promoting substance in chlorella was found consist of manganese and five chemically-active organic substances, one of them containing sulfur. One scientist ran an experiment to see if manganese alone was responsible for lactobacillus growth. He added manganese a little time to the lactobacillus growth medium, and the bacteria multiplied more th usual, but only 10% as much as when CGF was added. Manganese alone co not be responsible for the growth of lactobacillus or of the many other microorganisms, plants, animals and people whose growth is stimulated by chlorella. There had to be one or more active growth-promoting substances besides manganese.

We should realize that in man, manganese is found in the highest concentrations in the bones, liver, pancreas and pituitary gland, the "master gland" of the endocrine system. Manganese is the memory element and whe is deficient, the loss of memory associated with aging begins. Manganese is needed for the metabolism of protein, carbohydrates and fats and may play a important part in blood formation. Manganese is needed by the nerves, by th brain and for production of the sex hormones, as well as for the growth of bones. It is important to the body in many ways. We do not underestimate th importance of the trace element manganese in the chemistry and metabolism the body, but there is much more to CGF than manganese.

The sulfur-containing substance in CGF has been identified as a nucleotide-peptide complex. Chlorella is 3% RNA and 0.3% DNA, and CGI concentrated in these nucleic acids. The sugars of the nucleotide include glucose, mannose, rhamnose, arabinose, galactose and xylose. Amino acids i the peptide include gluta-mine, alanine, serine, glycine, proline, and asparag (Various researchers add threonine, lysine, cysteine, tyrosine, and leucine.) The molecular weight is less than 15,000.[29]

---

[28]*Bunso Rei, **Health Revolution,*** Nisshosha Co., Lt., Kyoto, Japan (undated translation from Japanese), p.5.

[29]*Ibid.*

It would be difficult to describe the many highly technical experiments scientists have run to find out what biologically-active substances are in CGF and what these substances do, singly and in combination. We must realize, however, that the reason why many scientists are putting so much time and effort into investigating chlorella and CGF is because there is already a great deal of proof that chlorella and CGF, even in relatively small amounts, stimulate growth, tissue repair and healing to an extent not previously found in any other food.

Particularly, experiments with young animals still in the growing stage have conclusively demonstrated that 1-5% addition of chlorella to the basic diet has promoted growth about 20%. In experiments with babies and children, amounts smaller than 1% have been associated with growth greater than that of controls, but not the 20% shown in animal experiments. In any case, results like these can't be explained by the amino acid content alone, or by the vitamins and minerals in chlorella. The same conclusion can be drawn from the healing, protecting, supporting effects of chlorella in regard to many organs, tissues and systems of the body.

In my travels around the world, searching for the secrets of health and long life, I found out that the foods people eat have a great deal to do with youthfulness, the repair and rebuilding of tissue, and a long, healthy life. When I visited Charlie Smith in Bartow, Florida, he was 135 years old, healthy, clear-minded and with a wonderful memory. It nearly blew my mind to find out he had been living the last 30 years on canned sardines and crackers! I wondered what could be in sardines to promote such health and longevity.

Then Dr. Benjamin Frank came out with his book, titled ***The No-Aging Diet***, showing that canned sardines were the highest-known food in RNA, one of the nucleic acids. Earlier he thought brewer's yeast was the highest RNA food, but then he found out sardines were 10 times higher. Chlorella is 10 times higher in RNA than sardines.

Eating foods high in nucleic acids provide the material for the repair and production of human nucleic acids, and it is the breakdown of DNA and RNA in the cells that is believed to be one of the main factors in aging and in degenerative diseases. I add, however, that both chlorella and sardines are *whole, pure and natural foods,* rich in trace elements. Sardines eat plankton, the tiny living sea organisms that convert sea minerals into living matter, organisms believed to be high in nucleic acids. Chlorella is grown in a "chemical soup" very much like sea water—rich in elemental nutrients dissolved in water.

Many seafoods have been found to be high in DNA (deoxyribonucleic acid), a complex molecule in the genetic material of each cell nucleus that contains the blueprint for the structure and function of the cell. In the cell nucleus, DNA forms RNA (ribonucleic acid) to act as cell "manager" and carry out all the instructions coded in the DNA for the life of the cell. When we eat foods high in DNA and RNA, the nucleic acids, they provide the basic materials for repair and replacement of our own DNA and RNA.

Seafoods are probably rich in nucleic acids because they grow in a relatively unpolluted, nutrient-rich environment, high in nearly all the basic chemical elements. With such a great variety of life forms available for fish lik sardines, anchovies and salmon, these fish became highest in the RNA factor. Measured in milligrams of RNA per 100 grams (3½ oz), fresh sardines have 343, anchovies 341 and salmon 289. Canned sardines, have 590 milligrams/10 grams, for reasons not understood, and it is the only fish higher in RNA canne than fresh. Chlorella has a remarkable 3 grams/100 grams of RNA.

They say that lobsters can live a hundred years or more, with no reductio in sex life at any time. Whales are long-lived, and so are sea turtles. The sea turtle is made up of nine different flavors of meat or flesh. How could the sea turtle have flavors like chicken, pork or beef as a sea animal? It is constantly bathed inside and out with seawater, and it lives on sea growth. The sea turtle is strong enough to carry an elephant on its back. It is a very healthy reptile, able to go a whole year without eating. I believe I see why the Mayans built temples to the turtles. For years, the French have made cosmetics using turtle oil to remove wrinkles and make the skin softer, more supple. Does turtle oil contain some factor that reverses the aging of the skin?

The long lives of some of the sea creatures may be due to their high RNA That's something to stop and think about.

Recent findings show that chlorella contains 3% RNA and 0.3% DNA, and of course, the liquid Chlorella Growth factor is a concentrated form of the nucleic materials. This means that chlorella has 5 times the amount of RNA as canned sardines, the food Dr. Frank found to be the highest in RNA. Of course, these findings on chlorella were not available at the time Dr. Frank wrote his book.

I want to say that I very much appreciate science and its many great discoveries, and I feel that science has begun to shed a little light on the mystery of Chlorella Growth Factor. I have the highest respect for the scientist of Japan, the Republic of China and many other nations that have investigated chlorella. But, sometimes nature does not reveal all her secrets. This is most obvious in the mystery of life itself, which science is unable to explain.

We know all of the nutrients, vitamins and minerals in chlorella. We kno how much chlorophyll is in it and what amounts of amino acids are there. We know something about its biologically-active components, and we know that the water-soluble material extracted from chlorella contains the substance responsible for growth and healing. We know very little, however, about the roles played by the various active substances in CGF as related to growth and healing. Do they work together or separately? Do they stimulate the brain or possibly the endocrine system?

One thing we know for certain. Everything scientists find out about chlorella increases our appreciation and admiration of it. When we think about the magic of sunshine energizing chlorophyll inside each tiny chlorella cell to create every substance in it, according to a genetic blueprint that is two billion years old, we can't help feeling overwhelmed by the mysterious power of good things in nature.

Chlorella is one of the greatest foods in nature, and one of the simplest, most primitive cells. Yet, science may never be able to unravel all of its extraordinary mysteries.

Is it possible that chlorella has a detoxifying effect much greater than scientists suspect? Is it possible that the Chlorella Growth Factor stimulates toxin-laden tissues to get rid of their toxins and then stimulates cell reproduction to rejuvenate the tissue, bringing in the new in place of the old?

Meanwhile, I am reminded of the Hunza people I met some years ago when I traveled to the Hunza Valley. These were possibly the healthiest people of the world at that time. Many of the men over 120 years of age still walked mountain trails daily to work in the fields. Their eyes were clear, they had every tooth in their heads and most had been sick only once or twice in their lives, if ever. They breathed pure mountain air, drank pure mountain water and ate mostly pure, whole, natural foods grown in rich soil and a little meat occasionally. They were simple people who knew nothing about vitamins, minerals, exercise or nutritionally-balanced meals. They didn't have to know. They were living close to nature and nature's principles without thinking or worrying about it.

While it is natural for us to wonder what chlorella is made of and why it has such a wonderful health-promoting effect on the body, we don't really need to know these things in order to use it. We know from studies, from experiments and the experiences of many people that chlorella protects the body from disease and often reverses diseases and restores health, without undesirable side effects.

We can say that some of the mystery of Chlorella Growth Factor has been unraveled, and at the same time, we can be glad that some mystery is left. It is possible that there will always be a little mystery in all healing.

21. BACK TO THE FUTURE

I feel that not only does chlorella draw us to natural principles of ıling, but it draws us into the future to help us adapt to the technological ͤ we live in. Chlorella is a realistic aid to better health in an era when ıdequate diet, stress and pollution contribute greatly to the deterioration of ılth in so many people.

In ages past, the topsoils of the earth were deep and fertile, the air and ter were pure and clean, and food crops were whole, pure, natural and, the most part, very nourishing. People walked more, worked harder ysically and lived healthier lives.

Not only was chlorella not needed, but the technology to grow and ocess it was not available until recent years.

Every great discovery, every great invention, seems to await that tain moment in history when a great need or crisis arises.

Over the past century, topsoils have diminished in fertility and depth. The centuries have taken their toll on the world's farmlands through erosion and over-production. Chemical fertilizers and pesticides are used all over the world. As pollution of the air, land and water has increased, food quality has decreased. With the arrival of the technological age, high-speed, high-stress living has become an accepted lifestyle for many. The great need of our age is a natural food supplement that balances and cleanses the body and helps protect against disease. Chlorella is an idea whose time has come.

We find that the same industrial, technological age that brought us so much of the pollution in this world, also brought out chlorella, which may be the most effective natural cleansing and protective food known to man. Chlorella can't be grown and processed properly without the help of modern technology. It may be that chlorella can be taken with prescription drugs, when they are necessary, to reduce or prevent dangerous side effects. It is ossible that chlorella may carry off the toxic residues of drugs, increasing the safety of prescription medication. This would be a great victory for the health arts.

One day, man will learn that we must live in harmony with nature, not in opposition to it. Then we will see a great restoring work being done on this planet, a time of cleaning up toxic waste and of returning to a more natural way of life.

Until that day comes, chlorella is one of the most effective foods in protecting us against toxic effects of pollution.

Chlorella is truly a "natural food:" Whole, pure and natural, not synthesized in a laboratory or processed so that many valuable nutrients are lost or so indigestible that we can't get much good out of it. Sun Chlorella's patented process for breaking down the cell wall makes its chlorella 80% digestible. People live at such a fast pace of life these days that they are constantly depleting their bodies of essential nutrients. Chlorella is the kind of food supplement we need to make up for these deficiencies. It is entirely without harmful side effects. Chlorella is one of the safest foods I know.

Chlorella builds and protects the body in many ways. Mr. Nakayama, now president of Sun Chlorella, was told by his doctor he had only a short time to live because a number of chronic diseases—including cancer—had reduced his health to the danger point. After taking chlorella, he "outlived" all his diseases. They are gone, he is still here, enjoying life. That's what caused him to get involved in chlorella development and production.

WE NEED "WHOLE BODY" FOODS LIKE CHLORELLA

Chlorella affects the whole body, rather than working specifically on a single disease. When the whole body is taken care of, it gains enough strength to throw off a disease in its own way, nature's way, without undesirable side effects, cumulative effects, time-bomb effects or abnormal genetic effects.

About 50 years ago, many doctors were concerned with proper nutrition. Interest faded as other therapies, such as drug therapy and surgery, became the proper thing. Now interest in nutrition is stirring again. I see a return of interest to what can be accomplished with food and natural nutrition. I believe more doctors every day are becoming interested in preventive medicine.

When we take chlorella, we reap certain specific benefits. We experience greater functional ability. The body is cleansed of toxic materials. We raise the level of immune system function, and cell membranes are strengthened. Building blocks for repair of our cellular nucleic acids are provided, and some mineral deficiencies are taken care of. Cell communities are strengthened, and tissue regains its integrity, especially as acids in the body are neutralized.

Every organ of the body is important in the proper functioning of every other organ and tissue, and this is a vital fact to consider as we try to understand how to build health and prevent disease. Just as one seriously impaired, underactive organ can drag down the functioning of all others, leading into a disease, so strengthening every organ and system in the body can lift the functional level of an organically impaired, underactive organ, leaving the disease behind. This is the way chlorella works.

Nutrition isn't everything in taking care of your body, but without nutrition, every other form of therapy is virtually worthless.

PROVEN WORTH—YOU CAN BANK ON IT!

Chlorella has demonstrated its effectiveness as a health builder, apparently regardless of the adequacy of the diet. In many testimonials presented in this book, I did not have access to information on the food habits of those whose diseases were left behind. They used chlorella tablets or chlorella tablets together with Chlorella Growth Factor. I don't know what they ate. Some may have had good diets, some may have had poor diets. We can't tell. What we know is that chlorella helped all of them.

I believe chlorella may be exactly the right supplement at the right time in man's history to make up for global food deficiencies and lift the health level of all mankind. It's an idea worth thinking about and acting upon.

Doctors talk about "broad-spectrum" drugs, drugs that are able to take care of a considerable number of condition. Chlorella is, similarly, a broad-spectrum supplement, able to lift the health level and assist the body in overcoming a variety of serious chronic diseases. It has established a very strong record in the past few years, both in scientific experiments with laboratory animals and in the experiences of thousands of people, showing great effectiveness against my disease conditions.

The traditional Japanese symbol for "medicine" carries the symbol for "food," "plants" or "forest," along with the symbol for "happiness."

This gives the idea that food should be our medicine, since the Japanese character literally means "enjoyment of the plant." This is the direction we should be going when considering our prospective on health and well-being. Man is part of nature, and when man and nature are in harmony, disease does not manifest. When man is out of harmony with nature, when disease symptoms appear, this is a sign of the need to look to nature for healing. I believe in this idea very much.

My travels in search of the understanding of chlorella have been a wonderful adventure for me. This great health treasure of the Orient becomes more interesting and more useful the more we learn about it. This has been quite an awakening for me, and I am very pleased to be able to share my discoveries with you. To me, chlorella is the "jewel of the Orient," one of the greatest health treasures of our time.

In all my travels and research, I haven't found a single case where this particular food, chlorella, is contraindicated. I have seen improvement in every patient of mine who used it. I am not talking about a cure. I look for foods and supplements that will take care of the whole body so that the body will cure itself.

My ambition has not been to become rich, famous or influential, but to bring out the greatest good possible in everyone I meet. I believe when you discover something good for mankind, it should be shared. This is the viewpoint of the teacher, an impersonal viewpoint, and I regard myself as a teacher more than anything.

I believe we will see chlorella used in our space programs of the future. I believe we will see it used to save the lives of premature babies. I believe we will be using chlorella to strengthen the immune system of those patients who are so depleted in energy that they can no longer resist the degenerative processes of disease. I believe we are only seeing the beginning of many useful future applications of chlorella.

Chlorella is moving into its proper place in the health arts with a useful role to fulfill. As a water plant, it takes in those chemical elements which it is genetically programmed to transform into nucleic factors, growth factors, vitamins, minerals, enzymes, protein, starches and fats—all useful, health-building substances. It transforms inorganic chemicals into bio-organic food.

This is a food that belongs in the consciousness of man. Every doctor, every hospital, should be interested in giving the best natural aids possible for getting patients well.

My only hope and sincere wish is that the path of your life will be better because of the values of chlorella shared in this book.

If I can be a blessing to you through my travels and my findings about chlorella, then I have done a good job.

THE DIGESTIBILITY AND BIO-AVAILABILITY STUDIES OF CHLORELLA

A partial translation from the, *"The Basic Studies And Applications Of Chlorella,"* by Takechi Yoshiko, Ph.D., of the Studying Research Center, Japan 1970.

EXPERIMENT

Chlorella samples used in the study were obtained from the mass cultivation in the open pond and were dried using various drying methods. The testing samples were mixed in the animal feeds and all adjusted to contain a 10% protein. Four wister rats (about 50 grams body weight) were given the testing samples for eight days, and the digestibility and bio-availability were determined according to the increase of body weights.

SUMMARY OF THE STUDY

The real digestibility was found higher than the previously reported data. The chlorella sample, dried with the lowest hot air gave 72% digestibility and the freeze dried sample gave 78%. The NaOH extract of protein from chlorella produced 76% digestibility. As the extracted protein was unable to exceed 60% from chlorella, the suitably dried chlorella samples would be adequate for digestibility study. As in previous experiments, chlorella samples with addition of methionine exceeded the bio-availability of casein. Based on the chronological experiments, the results of the digestibility data were compiled in Tables 5.62 and 5.63, for review.

CONCLUSION

1. Chlorella treated with different drying methods showed large differences only in the artificial digestibility test, but in the animal digestibility study, it showed no significant difference.

2. Decolorized chlorella with methanol increased the digestibility, but methanol is not allowed for human consumption.

3. The freeze dried chlorella sample showed an increase in the artificial digestibility test.

4. Samples with 10 minute wet heat treatment increased the digestibility, samples with a 2 minute treatment had questionable effectiveness.

5. The chlorella treated with different drying methods greatly affected the digestibility in the artificial tests. Samples dried with low temperature tended to increase digestibility.

6. In early studies, the spray dried samples seemed not to produce good digestibility. It was later found that spray drying using an efficient spray dryer or freeze drying were the most suitable drying methods.

7. Chlorella with cell wall crushed by mechanical means increased the rate of digestion in the artificial digestibility test.

8. The method of extracting protein from chlorella was not efficient, and its digestibility was not superior as compared to the whole chlorella. Hence, there is no necessity to make protein extract for digestion.

9. Chlorella without decolorization treated with suitable drying methods showed digestibility to 86%. This percentage is equal to that of beef liver and minced meat. Therefore, no digestibility problem should be concerned.

10. The bio-availability of chlorella with the addition of methionine exceeded casein.

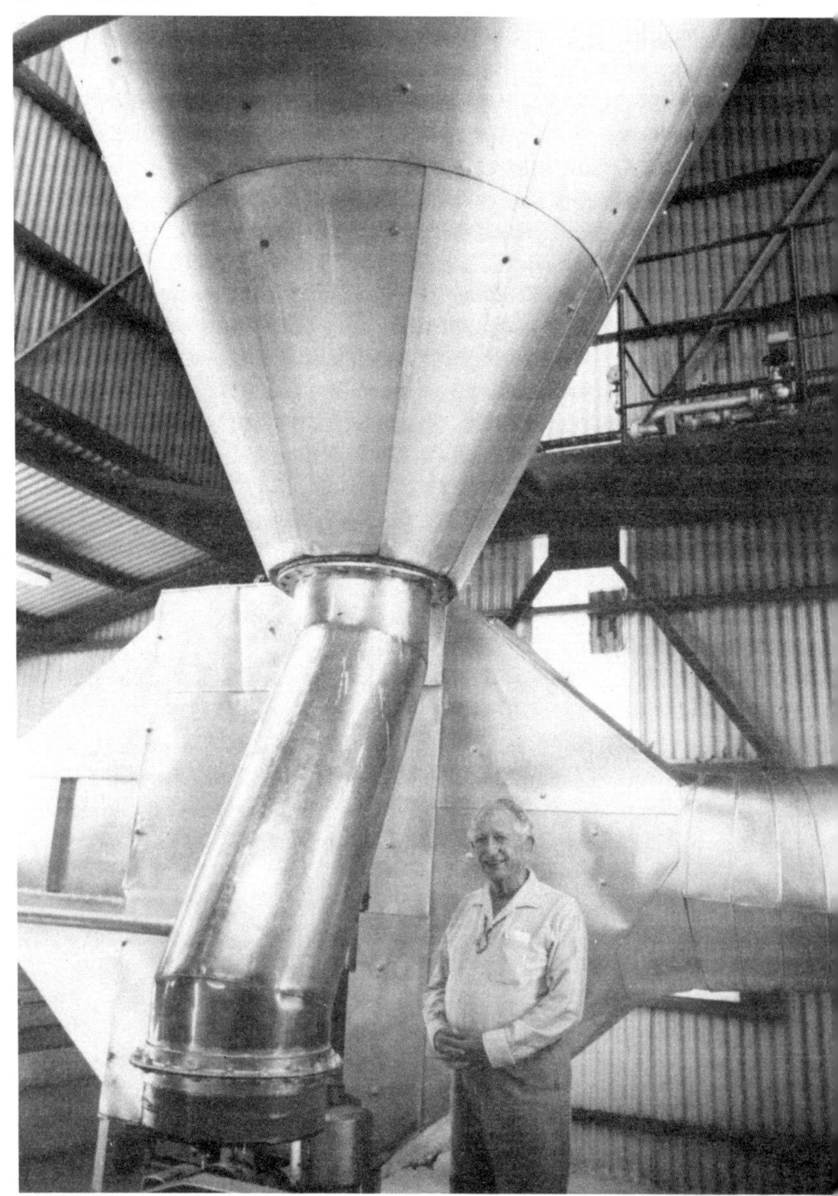

Table 5.62 **Digestibility and Bio-availability of the decolorized Chlorella and extracted protein from Chlorella**

Samples	Body Weight Increase	PER*	Apparent Digestibility	Real Digestibility	Bio-availability	NPU**
Decolorized Chlorella 20%	18.7	2.15	78.1	83.7	73.4	63.3
Decolorized Chlorella 10%	10.2	2.43	73.1	82.0	79.6	61.8
Same & Methionine	16.4	3.69	76.1	84.9	92.1	74.0
NaOH Extracted protein	9.0	2.29	77.5	86.7	81.3	67.4
Whole egg protein 20%	23.8	2.77	89.0	93.8	85.2	77.2
Same 10%	28.7	5.18	83.6	91.4	94.5	81.6
No protein	-5.5					
Decolorized Chlorella 10%	1.8	2.70	77.2	86.0	72.9	60.4

* PER Protein efficiency ratio
** NPU Net protein utilization

Table 5.63 **Digestibility and Bio-availability of the treated(different drying methods) Chlorella**

Samples	Body Weight Increase	PER*	Apparent Digestibility	Real Digestibility	Bio-availability	NPU**
Raw chlorella	24.0	3.24	62.5	74.5	89.6	66.7
Hot air dried Chlorella	6.4	1.55	58.9	72.3	72.7	52.6
Spray dried Chlorella	14.3	2.67	59.7	73.5	75.6	55.5
Freeze dried Chlorella	21.5	3.10	64.1	77.6	84.4	65.5
Decolorized Chlorella	14.5	2.56	70.8	84.8	84.6	71.8
Decolorized Chlorella and Methionine	31.8	3.71	71.8	84.9	90.8	77.1
NaOH Extracted protein from Chlorella	25.0	3.51	61.5	75.8	81.9	61.1
Casein	19.5	3.56	81.3	95.0	86.3	82.0
Whole egg protein	41.6	4.17	82.3	95.2	98.0	93.3
No protein	-7.9					

BIBLIOGRAPHY

1. Scientific Research Digest on Chlorella; Data Base: Medline; Range: 1/81 to 10/86; Capacity: 92; Medicinal Plant Institute of Hokkaido, Japan.
2. Schopf, J. William; "Precambrian Micro-Organism and Evolutionary Events Prior to the Origin of Vascular Plants," Biol. Rev. (1970), 45, pp. 319-352.
3. Kirk, R.E., and D.F. Othmer; Encyclopedia of Chemical Technology, Vol. 3, p. 879, The Interscience Encyclopedia, Inc., NY, 1949 (2nd ed.).
4. Gahan, E., P.R. Kline and T.H. Finkle; Chlorophyll in the Treatment of Ulcers. Arch Dermatol. Syphilol. 49, 849-851, 1943.
5. Hughes, J.H. and A.L. Latner; Chlorophyll and Haemoglobin regeneration after haemorrhage, J. Physiol. 86, 388-395, 1936.
6. Yamagishi, Y., Hasuda, S., Y. Mito, V. Experience in taking Chlorella for healing the less curable wound. In: Huang, C.J.: Application of Chlorella on Medicine and Food Technical Bulletin, March 1970. Taiwan Chlorella Manufacture Co., Ltd., Taipei, Taiwan.
7. Golden, T. and Burke, J.F.: Effective management of offensive odors. Gastroenterology, 31: No. 3, 1956.
8. Young, R.W. and J.S. Beregi. Use of Chlorophyllin in the Care of Geriatric Patients. J. Am. Geriatrics Soc. XXVIII, No. 1, p. 46-47, 1980.
9. Yoshida, A., et al., Gastroenterology Jpn 1980; 15(1); 49-61.
10. Manabe, T., et al., Ann. Surg. 190(1):13-7, Jul 1979.
11. Hagino, et al., Effect of chlorella on fecal and urinary cadmium excretion in "Itai-itai," Jpn J Hyg 30(1), 77, April 1975.
Biochem. 12. Northcote, D.H., K.J. Goulding and R.W. Horne, The Chemical Composition and Structure of the Cell Wall of Chlorella pyrenoidosa. J. 70:391-397, 1958.
13. Horikoshi, T., A. Nakamima and T. Sakaguchi: Uptake of Uranium by Various Cell Fractions of Chlorella regularis. Radioisotopes 28(8), 485-487, Aug. 1979.
14. Takechi, Yoshiro, "Chlorella—Its Basis and Application. Publ. by Gakushu Kenku-Sha, Tokyo, Japan, Nov. 30, 1971.
15. Yamaguchi, N., S. Shimizu, T. Murayama, T. Saito, R.F. Wang and Y.C. Tong: Immunomodulation by single cellular algae (Chlorella pyrenoidosa) and anti-tumor activities for tumor-bearing mice. Third International Congress of Developmental and Comparative Immunology, Reims, France, July 7-13, 1985.
16. Yamaguchi, N., S. Shimizu, T. Murayama, T.Saito, R.F. Wang and Y.C. Tong: Immunomodulation by single cellular algae (Chlorella pyrenoidosa) and anti-tumor activities for tumor-bearing mice. Presented at the Third International Congress of Developmental and Comparative Immunology, Reims, France, July 7-13, 1985.
17. Hixson, J.R., Beta-Carotene Showing Promise as Topical Agent., Medical Tribune, August 6, 1986, p.3.

18. Umezawa, I., K. Komiyama, N. Shibukawa, M. Mori and Y. Kojima: An Acidic Polysaccharide, chlon A, from Chlorella pyrenoidosa. Chemotherapy 30(9), 1041-1045, 1982.
19. Umezawal, I., K. Komiyama, N. Shibukawa, M. Mori and Y. Kojima: An acidic polysaccharide, chlon A, from Chlorella pyrenoidosa. Chemotherapy 30(9), 1041-1045, Sept. 1982. (in Jpn).
20. Shirota Minoru, et al. (Regarding the anti-virus components extracted from Chlorella.) Showa 42 nen Nihon nogika gakkai koen yori, 1967.
21. Kashiwa, Y. and Y. Tanaka: Effect of Chlorella on the changes in the body weight and rate of catching cold of the 1966 training fleet crew. Reported at the Japan Medical Science Meeting, Nagoya, Japan, 1966.
22. Umezawa, I., K. Komiyama, N. Shibukawa, M. Mori and Y. Kojima: An acidic polysaccharide, chlon A, from Chlorella pyrenoidosa. Chemotherapy 30(9), 1041-1045, Sept. 1982 (in Jpn).
23. Kollman, H.V. and R. Schmidt; Algae, The Modern Manna? Let's Live, December 1978.
24. Nomoto, K., T. Yokokura, H. Satoh and K. Mutai; Anti-tumor effect by oral administration of Chlorella extract. PCM-4. Gan-To-Kagaku-Ryoho, 10(3), 781-5, March 1983 (in Jpn).
25. Yamaguchi, N., S. Shimizu, T. Murayama, T. Saito, R.F. Wang and Y.C. Tong: Immunomodulation by Single cellular algae (Chlorella pyrenoidosa) and anti-tumor activities for tumor-bearing mice. Presented at the Third International Congress of Developmental and Comparative Immunology, Reims, France, July 7-13, 1985.
26. Lin, J-K., et al., Effect of Chlorella on Serum Cholesterol of Rats. Taiwan Medical Science Journal, Sept. 1981.
27. Sakuno, T., et al., Inhibitory effect of Chlorella on increases in serum and liver cholesterol levels of rats. Health Industry Newsletter, March 25, 1978.
28. Okuda, M., J. Hasegawa, M. Sonoda, T. Okabe, Y. Tanaka: The effects of Chlorella on the levels of cholesterol in serum and liver. Japanese J. Nutr. 33; 3-B, 1975.
29. Shimizu, M., N. Yamada, M. Hisada, J. Suzuki, I. Inata. Effect of Chlorella on Human Pulse Wave Velocity. Kanazawa Medical University, Dept. of Serology, April 8, 1985.
30. Hasuda, Shioichi and Y. Mito. Experience in taking chlorella for healing the less curable wound Chapter V. Application of Chlorella on Medicine and Food. Taiwan Chlorella Manufacture Co., Ltd., P.O. Box 1250, Taipei, Taiwan, 71, sec. 2 Nanking East Road, Taipi, Taiwan, R.O.C.
31. Krishnamurty, Goteti Bala. The Effect of Algae on Selected Bacterial Populations in Sewage, M.S. Thesis, UCLA 1959.
32. Taiwan Chlorella Manufacture Co., Ltd.; Application of Chlorella on Medicine and Food. Report Summaries, P.O. Box 1250, Taipei, Taiwan, 171, sec. 2 Nanking East Road, Taipi, Taiwan, R.O.C.

If You've Enjoyed Reading This Book . . .

Vibrant Health From Your Kitchen—One of Dr. Jensen's latest and greatest books. In this book, he teaches the basics of health and nutrition. A food guide for family health and well-being. The reader learns how proper foods can overcome certain mineral deficiencies, allergies and build immunity.

Food Healing of Man—Innumerable experiences are recounted in Dr. Jensen's work with both human beings and animals. The book is a comprehensive layman's guide to the healing power of foods elaborating on nutritional deficiencies. Lists 28 factors necessary for correcting body ailments. A study is made as to why foods heal and the reason for supplements.

Nature Has A Remedy—Solutions applying nature's restorative powers are discussed. A nature encyclopedia covering hundreds of ailments. Teaches methods of taking care of various symptoms encountered with diet, water treatments, physical exercise, climate, environment and others.

Tissue Cleansing Through Bowel Management—Toxic-laden tissues can become a breeding ground for disease. Elimination organs, especially the bowel, must be properly taken care of. This book tells the reader how. Bowel management through a balanced nutritional program with adequate fiber in the diet and regular exercise can often do wonders. A special 7-day cleanse will bring back energy, regenerate tissues and allow good food to let nature do its healing work.

The Healing Mind Of Man—The spiritual, mental and physical qualities of man must be considered for healing. All body functions depend upon our mind, and must be brought into balance before healing can occur.

A New Lifestyle For Health and Happiness—A concise summary of Dr. Jensen's most effective methods for restoring and maintaining good health. A sound program outlined with practical applications and daily charts for improving a person's lifestyle.

Vital Foods For Total Health, A Cook Book And Kitchen Guide—You are what you eat! Your health, your looks, and even the length of your life is affected by your diet. Your meals may look good and taste good, yet lack the vital elements your body requires. So to keep your health and your looks, or to regain them, eat correctly! This book will tell you how. This is a complete cookbook which combines health teaching and the newer knowledge of nutrition.

Foods That Heal—In the first half of this book, Dr. Jensen focuses on the philosophy and ideas of Hippocrates, the brilliant work of Dr. V. G. Rocine, and concludes with a look at his own pioneering work in the field of nutrition. The second half is a nutritional guide to fruits and vegetables.

For information on ***Dr. Jensen's Food Products for the 21st Century*** and for a ***free*** catalog of all his books and supplies, please write to:

Dr. Bernard Jensen
24360 Old Wagon Road
Escondido, CA 92027